Albert Duke

LOW-FODMAP DIET

A Step by Step Scientifically Proven Solution for Managing IBS and Other Digestive Disorders

TABLE OF CONTENTS

INTRODUCTION

For a layman, a FODMAP diet control instruction might provide a clue to some serious health issue, though it is not as serious as it sounds. The key concern is the malabsorption of natural sugars and carbohydrates that we eat every day in our food. Most people may be shocked, because nowadays diabetes problems have become one of the most common physical problems in people of all ages, particularly working young people.

The problem of bloating, stomach pain, and diarrhea rises every day in humans. If you have the issue of bloating after you eat, then now is the time to be vigilant with your food. When you are taking vegetables, fruits, and whole grains, you have the same problem. You remove the milk products from your diet to solve the problem, but the blowing continues to cause discomfort.

Bloating the stomach is frequently caused by anxiety but often by bad food choices. Following the Fodmap Dietary Plan, you can learn which foods bloat the intestines and are to be avoided and which foods will promote faster free digestion. This dietary plan is easy to use and gives anyone with a bloated stomach great relief from consuming the wrong foods. This is a normal means of healthy digestion without the need for antacids and other anti-bladder drugs.

CHAPTER ONE

What is FODMAP?

Food is a common digestive cause. Limiting some foods in susceptible people can significantly improve these symptoms.

In the treatment of irritable bowel syndrome, a diet known as FODMAPS is clinically recommended (IBS).

This book discusses how the diet of low FODMAP works and who should try it.

What is FODMAP?

What does FODMAP mean?

FODMAP means fermentable oligosaccharides, disaccharides, monosaccharides, and polyols that are short-chain carbohydrates (sugars), which are poorly absorbed through the small intestine. After eating them, some people suffer stomach discomfort. Symptoms are as follows:

- Diarrhea
- Cramping
- Stomach bloating
- Constipation
- Gas and flatulence

This is clinically known for classifying classes of carbs known to cause digestive symptoms such as bleeding, gas, and stomach pain.

FODMAPs are present in varying quantities in a wide variety of foods. Some foods contain only one type, and others contain more than one type.

The key dietary sources of the four FODMAP groups are:

Oligosaccharides: Rye, wheat, legumes, and other vegetables and fruit, such as onions and garlic.

Disaccharides: soft cheese, milk, and yogurt. Lactose is really the main carb.

Monosaccharides: Various fruits like mangoes and figs and sweeteners, including sweet nectar and honey. The key carbohydrate is fructose.

Polyols: certain fruit and vegetables, including blackberries and lychee, and some sweeteners with low calories such as gum free from sugar.

SUMMARY: FODMAPs are the group of fermentable carbohydrates that intensify intestinal symptoms in sensitive people. They are present in several foodstuffs.

Benefits of A Low-FODMAP Diet

High-FODMAP foods are limited in a low-FODMAP diet.

The advantages of a low FODMAP diet have been evaluated in more than 30 studies in thousands of people with IBS.

Reduced Digestive Symptoms

IBS symptoms can vary extensively, including reflux, bloating, stomach pain, flatulence, and bowel discomfort.

Stomach pain is a hallmark of the disease, and more than 80 percent of IBS patients have been found to be bloated.

These signs may, of course, be weakening. One major study also said people with IBS would give up an average symptom-free of 25 percent of their remaining lives.

Fortunately, both stomach pain and bloating with a low FODMAP diet has been shown to decrease significantly.

Data from four quality studies have shown that if you adopt the low-FODMAP diet, there is an 81% and 75% higher risk of improving bloating and stomach pain.

Several additional studies have shown that diet can lead to flatulence, diarrhea, and constipation.

Increased Quality of Life

People with IBS also show a decreased quality of life and associated extreme digestive symptoms.

Fortunately, numerous studies have shown that the low-FODMAP diet enhances overall life quality.

Some evidence also shows that a low-FODMAP diet can increase people's energy levels with IBS, but that placebo-controlled studies are required to support this finding.

SUMMARY:

The benefits of a low-FODMAP diet are compelling. In nearly 70 percent of adults with IBS, the diet tends to improve digestive symptoms.

Who Should Follow a Low-FODMAP Diet?

Not everybody has a low-FODMAP diet. If IBS is not diagnosed, the literature indicates that the diet will do more harm than good.

Since most FODMAPs are prebiotics, they help the growth of healthy intestinal bacteria.

Most research was also performed on adults. Therefore, in children with IBS, diet support is minimal.

Consider this diet if you have IBS:

- Continued gut symptoms.

- Has not responded to strategies for stress management.
- Haven't listened to the advice of the first line, like alcohol, caffeine, spicy foods, and other popular food causes.

That said, some speculation exists that the diet can support other conditions, including diverticulitis and digestive problems caused by exercise. Further analysis is continuing.

It is important to note that the diet is a mechanism involved. It is not advised to try it for the first time during a journey or during a busy or stressful period.

SUMMARY:

For adults with IBS, a low-FODMAP diet is recommended. The evidence for its use in other situations is restricted and more negative than nice.

How to Follow the Low-Fodmap Diet?

A diet with low FODMAPs is more complex than you think and consists of three levels.

Stage 1: Restriction

In this step, all high-fODMAP foods are strictly avoided. If you don't know which foods in FODMAPs are big.

People who adopt this diet frequently assume that all FODMAPs should be avoided in the long term, but that should take only around 3-8 weeks. This is because FODMAPs should be used in the gut health diet.

Some people see symptoms improvement in the first week, while others take eight weeks in full. You will proceed to the second stage once you have sufficient relief from your digestive symptoms.

If your intestinal symptoms have not improved for eight weeks, related to What Do Your Symptoms Not Improve? Below chapter.

Stage 2: Reintroduction

This stage includes reintroducing high FODMAP foods systematically.

The aim is double:

1. In order to classify which FODMAP forms you tolerate. Few are sensitive to them all.

2. You can tolerate deciding the amount of FODMAPs. This is called your "threshold level."

In this stage, you are checking those foods one by one for three days.

This move should be taken with a professional nutritionist who can direct you through the necessary foods. The app will also help you to classify which foods you want to reintroduce.

It should be noted that a low-FODMAP diet should be continued during this point. Even if a certain high-FODMAP food can be tolerated, you must continue to limit it until phase 3.

It is essential to note that people with IBS can withstand small quantities of FODMAPs, unlike most people with food allergies.

Finally, although digestive symptoms can weaken, they do not cause the long-term body harm.

Step 3: Personalization

This process is also known as the "modified FODMAP diet." In other words, some FODMAPs are still being limited. The sum and the form are, however, adjusted to your personal tolerance, as seen in stage 2.

To increase dietary variety and versatility, it is important to progress to this final point. This is related to better compliance over the long term, quality of life, and intestinal health.

SUMMARY:

Many people are shocked to see a three-story diet with low FODMAP. Each process is also essential to the long-term relief of symptoms and overall health and well-being.

THREE THINGS TO DO BEFORE YOU GET STARTED
Before you start your diet, there are three things you should do.

1. Make sure you've got IBS.

Digestive symptoms can be more pronounced in many, some harmless and others.

Sadly, no positive diagnostic test is available to confirm that you have IBS. It is as well as best to consult a doctor first to exclude more extreme disorders, such as coeliac, inflammatory bowel disease, and colon cancer.

Once excluded, the doctor will confirm that you have IBS using the official IBS diagnostic criteria — you need to follow all three to obtain an IBS diagnosis:

• Chronic stomach pain: On average, in the last three months, at least one day a week.

• Stool symptoms: there are two or more: defecation related, associated with a change in stool frequency, or with a change in stool appearance.

• Persistent symptoms: guidelines met over the last three months with the onset of symptoms not less than six months prior to diagnosis.

2. Try Diet Methods First Line

The low FODMAP diet is a time-consuming process.

Therefore, it is considered second-line dietary guidance in clinical practice and is only used in a subset of IBS-persons that do not respond to first-line strategies.

3. Plan Ahead

If you are not prepared, the diet can be difficult to obey. Here are a few tips:

• See what to purchase: make sure that you have access to credible low-FODMAP food listings. See below for a list of places.

• Remove high FODMAP food: remove your refrigerator and the dispenser.

Make your shopping list: Build a low-FODMAP shopping list before you go to the grocery store so that you know which food to buy or stop.

• Read menus in advance: get to know low FODMAP menu choices so that you're ready to dine.

SUMMARY:

There are many items you must do before you start the low-FODMAP diet. These easy measures help improve your ability to control your digestive symptoms effectively.

A LOW-FODMAP DIET CAN BE FLAVORFUL

In FODMAPs, garlic and onion are both very strong. This contributed to the widespread belief that there was no taste in a low-FODMAP diet.

Although many recipes make use of onion and garlic, many low-FODMAP herbs, spices, and savory flavors can be substituted.

We should also emphasize that the taste of garlic can still be obtained using strained garlic-infused oil, which is low in FODMAPs.

It is because the FODMAPs in the garlic were not fat-soluble, which means that the flavor of garlic is transferred to oil, but the FODMAPs are not transferred.

Suggestions for the Low-FODMAP are chives, chili, fenugreek, ginger, citrus fruit, mustard, pepper, Safran, and turmeric.

A more detailed list could be found here.

Summer:

There are many common FODMAP flavors, but many low-FODMAP herbs and spices can be used to make delicious foods.

CAN VEGETARIANS FOLLOW A LOW-FODMAP DIET?

A healthy vegetarian diet in FODMAPs can be poor. However, if you are a vegetarian, a low-FODMAP diet can be more difficult.

High FODMAP legumes are the staple protein foods in the vegetarian diets.

That said, small portions of rinsed and canned legumes can be included in a low-FODMAP diet. Portions are usually roughly 1/4 cup (64 grams).

There are also several protein-rich low-FODMAP choices for vegetarians, including tofu, tempeh, quorn, eggs, and most nuts and grains.

Summer:

There are several vegetarian protein-rich choices for low-FODMAP diets. There is no reason, therefore, why an IBS vegetarian cannot adopt a well-balanced low-FODMAP diet.

A LOW-FODMAP SHOPPING LIST

Many foods in FODMAPs are naturally low.

Here is an easy list to start shopping.

- Protein: meat, poultry, chickens, fish, lamb, swine, cream, and tofu.
- Whole grains: Brown rice, buckwheat, maize, millet, quinoa, and oats

- Outflow: bananas, blackberries, kiwi, lime, mandarin, orange, papaya, ananas, rhubarb, and strawberries
- Vegetables: Bean spruces, bell peppers, carrots, choy sum, aubergine, kale, onions, spinach, and courgettes.
- Nuts: almonds (no more than 10 per seat), peanuts, peanuts, pines, and walnuts.
- Seeds: lens, pumpkin, sesame, and sunflower
- Dairy: Cheddar cheese, Parmesan, and lactose-free milk
- Oils: Olive oil and coconut oil.
- Beverages: black tea, coffee, green tea, mint tea, water, and white tea
- Condiments: basil, chili, ginger, mosquito, pepper, salt, vinegar, white rice, and wasabi Pulver

In addition, it is important to review the list of ingredients for additional FODMAPs in packaged foods.

For many reasons, for example, as prebiotics, as a fat substitute, or as a lower calorie the substitute for sugar, food companies may add FODMAPs to their foodstuffs.

Summer:

Many foods in FODMAPs are naturally tiny. Many processed foods have added and should be limited to FODMAPs, therefore.

What if your symptoms cannot be improved?

The low-FODMAP diet does not work with IBS at anyone. Around 30% of people do not respond to the diet.

Fortunately, other non-dieting treatments can aid. Speak about alternative solutions to your doctor.

That said, you should: before you give up the low-FODMAP diet

1. Lists of ingredients search and check

Prepackaged foods also have secret FODMAP origins.

Onion, garlic, sorbitol, and xylitol are widely considered to cause symptoms even in limited quantities.

2. Consider your FODMAP information's accuracy

There are several online low-FODMAP food lists.

However, only two universities offer comprehensive, validated FODMAP food and app lists.

3. Think Other Stressors of Life

Diet isn't the only thing which can make the symptoms of IBS worse. Another big cause is stress.

Indeed, no matter how effective your diet is, your symptoms are likely to continue if you are under extreme stress.

Summer:

The low FODMAP diet is not ideal for all. However, it is worth testing common errors before pursuing other therapies.

What should I eat on the diet of FODMAP?

How does the low diet of FODMAP work?

Low FODMAP is a 3-stage disposal diet:

First, you stop eating any foods (high FODMAP foods).

Next, you reintroduce them slowly to see which of them are disturbing.

Once you recognize foods that cause symptoms, you can avoid or limit them while you are restless.

"We recommend only 2 to 6 weeks after the elimination portion of the diet," says Veloso. "It will reduce the symptoms and help decrease abnormally high intestinal bacteria if you have SIBO. Then every three days, you should add a high FODMAP diet, one at a time, to see if it causes symptoms. If a high FODMAP food triggers symptoms, avoid that long-term."

Foods that because symptoms differ between people.

In order to ease IBS and SIBO symptoms, it is important to avoid the high FODMAP foods, including:

The Dairy-based milk, ice cream, and yogurt
Wheat based products include bread, cereal, and crackers.

Beans and lentils
Some vegetables include asparagus, artichokes, onions, and garlic.
Certain fruits include cherries, apples, peaches, and pears.

Basis your food around low FODMAP foods like:

Meat and eggs
Some cheeses like Camembert, brie, feta, and cheddar

Almond milk
Grains such as quinoa rice and oats
Vegetables such as potatoes, eggplant, cucumbers, tomatoes, and zucchini
Fruit include oranges, pineapple, grapes, blueberries, and strawberries,
Get your doctor or nutritionist with a complete list of FODMAP foods.

Who should try it?

The low FODMAP diet for the IBS and SIBO is part of the treatment. Research has shown that symptoms are decreased in up to 86% of people.

Because the first, most restrictive step of the diet can be daunting, it is crucial to work with a doctor who can ensure that you follow the diet properly—which is critical for success—and maintain correct nutrition.

"This should not be tried on its own by anyone who is underweight," said Veloso. "The low FODMAP diet is not intended to lose weight but can lose weight since too many foods are eliminated. For someone who is still too fragile, it can be risky to lose more."

How can a doctor help?

Dietary modifications may have a significant effect on symptoms of IBS and SIBO, but physicians may often use other therapies. Antibiotics can rapidly eliminate minor bacterial overcrowding, whereas laxatives and low-dose bowel syndrome can ease symptoms.

The best approach is always a mix of lifestyle modifications, treatments, and stress management strategies. Learn how you can find SIBO and IBS therapies that work well for you with a doctor.

FODMAP Intolerance, The Problem and Solution to Control It

To a layman, a FODMAP diet control guidance may suggest a serious health condition, but it is not as serious as it sounds. The key concern stems from the malabsorption of natural sugars and carbohydrates that are present in the foods that we eat every day. This may surprise most people because nowadays, the diabetes problem has come to be one of the most common physical problems in people of all ages, particularly among working young people.

Ok, I want to hear something from you people before I go ahead. Do you know that your sugar-free dairy is enriched with natural sugar and carbohydrates as a balanced diet, and even the fruit you eat every day are also enriched with sugar and carbohydrates? If for whatever cause, your body cannot even digest or absorb these foods, you are asked to limit your FODMAP diet. The signs of this problem are very common and can be found in bloating, nausea, stomach pain, constipation, etc.

What is the FODMAP acronym?

FODMAP is abbreviated in Fermentable, Oligosaccharides, Disaccharides, Monosaccharides, and Polyols.

They can be described further as:

- It is fermentable when sugar and carbohydrates are broken by the bacteria in the wide bowl.
- This is a mixture of two terms, "oligo" and "saccharides," referring respectively to a few sugars. They are usually the mixture of various sugar molecules.
- Disaccharides, apply to molecules of double sugar.
- Monosaccharides, referring to the single sugar molecule.
- Polyols that apply to sugar alcohols.

How do FODMAP items build physical problems?

If a person's small intestine cannot consume sugar and natural carbohydrates, they pass into the big intestine and trigger problems:

The products of FODMAP are fermented by the bacteria in the broad bowel that leads to the appearance of gas.

The wide bowl draws water in the second case.

These situations lead to issues such as bloating, stomach pain, dehydration, constipation, etc.

How to control the FODMAP problem?

The issue of malabsorption can be solved, as mentioned above, by reducing the amount of FODMAP products in their daily diets. But the problem for most people is that they hesitate to talk about the problem before others, even before doctors. It is best to speak to the doctor about the issue without hesitation. After diagnosing the reasons for the emergence of your problem, two phases of treatment will be recommended.

Is the FODMAP Diet Behind the Problem of Bloating or Diarrhea?

In humans, the issue of bloating, stomach pain, and diarrhea grows regularly. If you have the issue of bloating after meals, now is the time to pay attention to your diet. When you take vegetables, fruit, and whole grains, the same issue arises. To fix the problem, the milk products have been eliminated from your diet, but there is no change.

Sometimes the food you have had in the morning triggers issues in the evening diet. It pulls you into a tangle. You don't know what kind of food the problem is making. What if, after going to the bathroom, you felt better? If you have diarrhea or shift a little, you feel relaxed when you come back from the bathroom, but with time. It may be FODMAP intolerance if you go through one of these stages. The FODMAP diet your digestive tract can tolerate needs to be monitored.

Doctors typically prescribe food containing low-FODMAP. Ok, don't mistake the name. It's not a serious illness or a very dangerous term. It is just a short name for many kinds of carbohydrates found in food. They are available in fruit, grain, and vegetable varieties.

It stands for fermentable oligosaccharides, disaccharides, monosaccharides, and polyols that are also sub grouped. The name displays only fermentable ones as the name suggests in the first letter 'F.' Disaccharides, for example, is the name of common sugar. But only one of several is fermentable, which can be contained in milk, i.e., lactose.

Most people find it difficult to absorb high FODMAP foods, especially oligosaccharides and polyols. And gastrointestinal disorders are the product. But if they're really low in their diet, they're not harmful and don't respond. However, very shortly after taking a small amount of these carbohydrates, people with SBI or other functional digestive disorders respond.

Besides, disaccharides and monosaccharides in healthy people do not cause any bad reactions. Lactose and fructose are the causes for the issue in both forms of carbohydrates. Yeah, the issue is that these carbohydrates are not digested throughout the broad intestine.

Amylase is the enzyme that helps to digest carbohydrates. This enzyme is produced in the mouth by chewing the food, moving through the digestive tract into the intestine. This mechanism breaks down the carbohydrates into the sugar that the cells consume and transfer energy across the body.

If the body is FODMAP intolerant, carbohydrates are not adequately digested in the small intestine and are unaccounted for by insufficient enzymes. Bacteria in the large intestine digest the sugars and cause functional gut disease symptoms.

CHAPTER TWO

Guidelines for Effective Dietary Management of Fructose Malabsorption: The Low FODMAP Diet

Sensitivity to sugars such as fructose, lactose, and sorbitol, but responsible for bloating the stomach and intestinal pain, too many, are mostly undiagnosed. The osmotic behavior and fast fermentation in the gastrointestinal tract have been demonstrated to be indigestible carbohydrates or sugars, like oligosaccharides, disaccharides, monosaccharides, and polyols. Various studies have shown that these sugars are a major cause of gastrointestinal symptoms in person or combined patients with fructose malabsorption and IBS.

The low FODMAP diet has significantly enhanced the gastrointestinal health of many people in clinical trials with fructose malabsorption and irritable bowel syndrome. FODMAPs represent the food types that are most vulnerable to intestinal bacteria fermentation. There is evidence that reducing the global FODMAP intake to treat functional gut symptoms offers relief for approximately 75% of FGD patients, such as irritable intestinal syndrome. Functional intestinal symptoms differ between individuals. Functional intestinal conditions are treated differently. Changes in meal size, alcohol, fat, and caffeine play a key role. Consumption of sufficient fiber and plenty of fresh, pure water also helps to track and sustain good digestive health dramatically. It is a must to consider the side effects of supplements and drugs. Changes to the lifestyle, including relaxation, exercise, good sleep, and sunshine, are also the main components of the Low FODMAP Diet.

This low-absorbed, short-chain carbohydrate group known as FODMAPs was developed by Australian researchers Dr. Sue Shepherd and Professor Peter Gibson. They coined the word FODMAP as a way of classifying some forms of carbohydrates as otherwise unrelated. The FODMAP acronym refers to fermentable oligosaccharides, disaccharides, and monosaccharides. It is used to describe a category of short-chain carbohydrate and sugar alcohols otherwise unrelated. The FODMAPs are fermented by bacteria that cause bloating, discomfort, reflux, diarrhea, and constipation of the intestines.

By reducing dietary FODMAPs, it is obvious that the majority of people with fructose malabsorption and those with irritable bowel syndrome have been effective in relieving these symptoms. Fructose is only one of many short-chain short, poorly absorbed carbohydrates that cause fructose malabsorption symptoms. There are complex names for a set of food molecules that some people poorly absorb. When these molecules are poorly absorbed in the small intestine, they serve as a source of food for digestive bacteria, leading to high osmotic activity and rapid fermentation and luminous dilution and resulting symptoms in those with less adaptable bowels or visceral hypersensitivity.

In individual fermentations of short-chain carbohydrates such as fructose and lactose, polyols are typically poorly absorbed, and fructus and galactans are often poorly absorbed in all. Food intake high in FODMAPs results in a rise in the amount of liquid and gas in the small and large intestines, leading to dislocation and symptoms such as abdominal pain, gas, and bloating.

Those with fructose malabsorption are significantly improved by the Low FODMAP diet. Many people have a better quality of life as a result of this diet. This diet includes a variety of dietary changes. Before beginning, consult a licensed nutritionist or dietitian to make sure you get the right nutrition, including fiber. It is also important to understand that FM can coexist with intolerance to other food chemicals such as additives, salicylates, amines, lactose, or gluten, so caution must be taken while you are still having symptoms in your diet. Studies (currently at the Monash University in Australia) on foods inside the FODMAP diet are still being performed. This diet is only in the early stages. New research will be exposed as time passes, and further experiments are carried out.

If the patient can handle such foods, it is up to the patient to find his own personal tolerance level. The Low FODMAP diet serves as a reference for this. Until now, no such guide has been published. Up to now, patients with fructose malabsorption and IBS have blindly understood what they can and cannot eat. Many foods have no immediate effect on the patient, so symptoms will only occur days later. It can be very hard to know what causes the symptoms. Symptoms can start later days and end later. The loop that continually overrides itself ensures that patients are still symptomatic. The accumulative effect and the chemistry between FODMAPs is a key factor. You are a research laboratory walking. It takes some time to decide your own meal schedule. In the first week, many see changes. You would also like to purchase a notebook for a food report. Document all; every food, every drink, every drug, everything ingested, and of course, the times. Record all. You may want to log the symptoms and times. This helps you to recognize a pattern.

The dietary advice for reducing carbohydrate fermentation in the bowel differs for each person. You may minimize symptoms by reducing the amount of fermentation carbohydrates. In certain cases, small quantities of these carbohydrates are also tolerated. Total avoidance of a specific food, such as onions, is a must to improve symptoms. It is important to understand that foods with different FODMAP values can add up, leading to symptoms which you do not encounter if you consume the food alone. For example, fruits that contain excess the fructose combined with natural polyols, including apples and pears, would likely trigger more serious symptoms, as the excess content of fructose and polyols adds to the overall load of FODMAP. The FODMAP: fructose, fructans, lactose, polyols, e.g., raffinose and Galatians. (sorbitol and artificial sweetener).

Fructose: This is a single sugar that is widely known as fruit sugar. Lt's in fruit, lots of vegetables and a lot of other foods. In many industrial and manufactured goods, fructose is a popular additive.

Lactose: A sugar in most milk and milk products. Since FODMAPs collectively affect GI symptoms, it is best to reduce lactose intake. Breath testing of hydrogen can be performed. Many fruit products are intolerant to lactose because it is the most common allergy in the population. If you are uncertain, lactose should be avoided. Lactose sensitivity leads to abdominal bloating, pain, gas, and diarrhea, frequently occurring 30 to two hours after milk and milk products are ingested. Intolerance to lactose is not metabolized due to a lack of the enzyme lactase required in the digestive system. Seventy-five percent of adults around the world are estimated to experience some reduction in lactase production during adulthood. Lactose tolerance varies, and dietary management of lactose intolerance relies on specific levels of tolerance. Lactose is present as a food additive in two broad categories of food: traditional dairy products; (in dairy and nondairy products).

Lactose (also present when labels say lactoserum, whey, milk solids, changed milk ingredients, etc.) is a commercial dietary additive used in order to make it tasteful, textured, and adhesive. It can be found in foods like processed meats.

Fructans: Fructans are long fructose chains 'stuck' at the end, with a glucose molecule (polymerized fructose chain with terminal glucose). Wheat and some vegetables such as onion are the major dietary sources of fructans. Inulin or fructo-oligosaccharides are also recognized (FOS). Fructans are food for digestive tract bacteria. This triggers the effects of fructose malabsorption, and no glucose can make it easier to digest these fructose chains. It should be exclusively limited to fructans.

Polyols: Polyols are also referred to as sugar alcohols. They do not have calories and do not break down or digest at all in the body. Most of them are too big to simply diffuse from the small intestines, causing a gastrointestinal laxative impact. These include sugar alcohols named after sorbitol, manitol, maltitol, xylitol, and isomalt. Overuse can have a laxative effect. If all you had to eat was without fructose for three days, you would possibly have no signs of polyols. However, this is really difficult to do. Also, glucose-balanced fructose causes the chemical reaction of polyols within the body. In certain fruits and vegetables, polyols also occur naturally. They are also used as an artificial sweetener and are added to sugar-free gums, cough drops, mints, and drugs as a sweetener. Polyols induce malabsorption of fructose if the digestion is normally safe. FM signs are much greater for people who already have polyols for fructose malabsorption. This is because polyols make fructose absorption much harder. It is advisable to restrict or eliminate polyols together. Some fruits and vegetables with polyols can be eaten by different individuals with an individual tolerance. The lawyers are one example. Polyols can include apricots, strawberries, nectarines, cerries, plums, pears, mushrooms, and prunes.

Galactans: It is oligosaccharides that have sugar galactose chains that end in fructose and glucose. The human body did not have the enzymes to hydrolyze them into the digestible components, so they contribute fully to gas and GI pain. Examples of Galatians are processing and stachyose. These are found in vegetables, including peas, onions, and other vegetables (baked beans, lentils, chickpeas).

The Low FODMAP Diet: fructose malabsorption dietary control.

1. Food with elevated free fructose levels and 'short-chain fructans' avoidance.

2. Total fructose load is reduced.

3. Food recommendation with healthy levels of fructose and glucose.

4. Free glucose consumption.

5. Low FODMAP diet for 8 - 10 weeks. If there is a change, one by one, the individual component will be questioned. Set a personal level of tolerance for you. Note the accumulative impact of FODMAP in your body. It is recommended you pursue a dietitian's advice to make sure you get the right nutrient and fiber requirements.

High fructose food: High fructose foods with a higher percentage of fructose than glucose can cause various adverse reactions to those with fructose malabsorption. They should be stopped or strictly limited. Free glucose intake can help absorb excess fructose, but the amount of fructose the small intestine can tolerate still remains restricted. In general, fructose is a concern only when more fructose is present than glucose or too much fructose is ingested in a single location, such as consuming two or three fruits in one sitting. Some foods with high fructose are:

- Apples (all varieties)
- Honey
- Dried fruit
- Pears
- Corn syrup
- Coconut in any form

- Fruit juice
- Honeydew melon
- Peaches
- Watermelon
- High fructose corn syrup
- Lychee
- Star fruit
- Canned fruit
- Nashi fruit

Foods Containing Fructans:

- Wheat (in large quantities) Trace amounts of wheat, as compared to celiac disease, are generally okay and well tolerated with FM.
- Rye (in large amounts)
- Brown rice: Many record brown rice difficulty. It can be ideal in small quantities.
- Onions (all varieties), even though consumed in small quantities, are the Main concern.
- Dandelion tea
- Zucchini
- Leeks
- Inulin (artificial fiber added to foods etc. Check labels.)
- Chicory
- Fructo-oligo saccharides (FOS) (artificial fiber added to some foods)
- Artichokes

Foods Containing Sorbitol:

- Artificial sweeteners: Mannitol, Sorbitol. Isomalt, Xylitol.

- Artificially sweetened gum, soft drinks and candy
- Apricots
- Apples
- Cherries
- Apricots
- Peaches
- Pears
- Nectarines

Foods Containing Raffinose:
- Brussel sprouts
- Cabbage
- Asparagus
- Baked beans
- Legumes
- Green beans, Red kidney beans
- Chickpeas
- Lentils

Lactose is found in most dairy foods, some more so than others. The following are at the top of the continuum.

Foods Containing High Levels of Lactose:
- Milk
- Ice cream
- Soft cheeses
- Condensed milk

Necessity of the Hydrogen and Methane Breath Test

If you'd enjoy food, you'd have no chance of eating your favorite food excessively at home, party, or on the market and would not have faced various forms of digestive issues the next day after you woke up. Well, this problem is not only connected with you, but it has recently become one of the common problems for all those sitting next to you. So the question that now arise as to why everybody has this problem. To answer that question, you should first realize that excess is always unhealthy and the same concept when you are consuming your favorite dish in excess.

The food we consume consists of different types of sugars that, apart from improving the taste of foods, also strengthen our immune system, but if the consumption of excess sugars starts to cause various types of stomach problems such as discomfort, gastric, bloating, etc. To get rid of this problem, you have to undergo a hydrogen and methane test, which allows you to diagnose the problem and find the appropriate remedy so that your beloved dish can be enjoyed without fear next time. Here, it should be held in mind that people with poor digestive systems would more likely be caught up in this dilemma, mainly because their stomach's food absorption efficacy is not high.

When we speak about the breath test to detect the appearance of hydrogen and methane in the body, we should know that it is a dangerous test, which can also be carried out at home, and its credentials can then be forwarded to the testing center for further examinations. There are various types of tests carried out to diagnose stomach disease, as follows:

1. Fructose Breath Test: to detect fructose sugar malabsorption;

2. Lactulose Breath Measure: Test hydrogen production in your stomach and gut transition time.

3. Lactose Breath Test: Excess lactose in the body to be checked.

4. Mannitol Breath Test: Detecting mannitol malabsorption.

5. Sorbitol Breath Test: Scan for Sorbitol malabsorption.

6. Sucrose Breath Test: Excess Sucrose malabsorption should be diagnosed.

Hydrogen and methane breath research methods:

As described above, during our daily activities, we take different types of sugar in our food in the form of fructose, lactose, sucrose, etc. As a general digestive procedure, these sugars go straight into our tiny stomach bowl. Individuals with low digestive efficiency cannot consume these carbohydrates, which causes sugar in a colon or large cup, which causes fermentation of unabsorbed sugars in the colon and produces a variety of gastrointestinal issues such as diarrhea, lack of appetite, bloating, irritable intestinal syndrome, etc.

During the breath test, it is diagnosed that either hydrogen or methane or the combination of both bacteria that has formed in the big bowl grow. The gas produced in the bowel transits in blood by the veins and comes out in the form of respiration by the lungs.

In some circumstances, it is found that patients do not suffer from the issue of generating hydrogen in excess of quantity; these patients are known as the "low producers of hydrogen" and, despite producing hydrogen, emit excess gas methane. It is also found that there are many patients who develop excess hydrogen but who develop methane because it metabolizes rapidly. Whatever the cause for this, patients with such problems have a negative hydrogen test and are told they have no malabsorption problem.

It is recommended to undergo a lactuose hydrogen test in order to solve such problems, which makes it easier for doctors to recognize the type of gas often created by bacteria. This test enables you to assess the time necessary for the transfer of sugar to your wide bowl during intake. Please bear in mind that this test is carried out to determine the absorption by our bodies of various sugars and their role in the emergence of problems such as bloating, wind and stomach pain, etc.

If positive signs are seen during the test, it is an indicator you can consume the specified percentage of the sugar prescribed for users. But, if the results of your breath tests are unfortunately negative, this does not mean that you should avoid using these sugars entirely; for such patients, there is a separate diet chart that favors the use of these sugars in a reduced percentage.

Discovering & Treating Dairy Sensitivity by an Elimination Diet

That's better said than done. Removal of milk items is far more than throwing out cheese dip, milk, ice cream, and most yogurts. Milk is listed in so many items in its entirety and component form.

It may be that what causes a person to be responsive to milk is one aspect of milk. Lactose is the most well-known part of milk that causes problems. People that are intolerant to lactose do not contain enough of the lactase enzyme used in digestion to break up lactose. This contributes to tension in the stomach, uncomfortable gas, flatulence, bloating, and/or stress in the stomach.

Intolerance to lactose primarily causes the same symptoms as milk sensitivities. Nausea, flatulence, and cramps have a common sensation, whether the reaction to milk is a consequence of a general allergy to cow's milk or lactose intolerance.

The signs of a full-blown dairy allergy should be remembered. Even if a dairy allergy can cause many of the same symptoms as both milk susceptibility or lactose intolerance, an allergy is an immune reaction that can run between two ends and can at any time alter the intensity of the reaction. A mild allergic reaction may be indigestion or a skin reaction such as hives. A severe reaction may also be caused by hives but may also be life-threatening as multiple organ systems are involved. The swelling symptoms can fully obstruct one's ability to breathe.

If you suspect sensitivity, it's time to begin reading labels! Look for ingredients such as whey, casein, and lactose that are milk or milk components. These words repeat themselves. Whey. Whey. Casein. Casein. Lactose. Lactose. Don't assume it is because a commodity is not generally considered to be even remotely associated with something that includes milk or its components. Whey and casein were used in so many processed foods that the list is too broad to include. Look at the label for something that sounds like milk, including words such as "cream," "butter," or "heavy cream," as well as the above-mentioned three red-flag words: whey, cashein, and lactose.

Now, you do not have to read every product label in your shops, and you don't have to learn every food ingredient on a restaurant menu. Read the labels and lists of ingredients for the food you eat. Be sure that, while eating, the server knows your dietary constraints and also asks if there is a dairy-free menu. Many of the bigger restaurant chains have milk-free choices. After you start your diet, as it is called, continue to look and learn on a regular basis what is consumed in the food.

When checking whether they are susceptible to a certain food, many fail to recognize three caveats. Many people who embark on an elimination diet to eliminate possible offending food will try to decide whether, after only a few days, they feel better or not. In order to give it a true shot, a minimum of a full month on the elimination diet is needed to see if symptoms change. Second, during the removal, many will test out some alternatives to milk. When you want to figure out if a certain food allergy is real, now is not the time to add new foods into your diet. New foods and alternatives to soy-based milk, which are another food that many people are very sensitive to, can contribute to allergy problems in people who are already sensitive to dairy products.

A diet for removal should be focused on keeping your daily diet minus the alleged perpetrator to discover whether you are susceptible to a suspected offending food product. If the symptoms begin to decline when milk is removed from the diet, the culprit is most likely to be milk. Finally, several people have multiple sensitivities, such as milk, ovum, or dairy and gluten, so the elimination diet often doesn't help, whether there is a dairy allergy, but only in combination with another food intolerance.

It is the best idea to take a thorough inventory of symptoms before initiating the elimination diet and to review symptoms for improvement every 1-2 weeks. After a few months on an elimination diet, the gut starts to heal, and some susceptible individuals can slowly and over time reintroduce milk. However, you should note that after years of symptomatic illness, it takes time to cure it, only after a reasonable period of time (at least three months) and slowly and cautiously. The reintroduction of milk in a sensitive individual may cause symptoms to recur or not. If symptoms recur, cut the milk again. If symptoms do not recur, it is still prudent to reduce the milk consumption indefinitely in order not to risk re-emergence.

For people who only must eat milk, although the symptoms are often almost intolerable, it's always your preference. Often signs are very tolerable depending on the type and the time of consumption of milk products. If the favorite cheese in the pizza is a must, and if the signs are just a little nausea and a bloated feeling, then it is maybe worthwhile for others to be uncomfortable eating the pizza. Just be conscious that the pain comes from something within your body that is wrong, and maybe the slight digestive symptoms are just the tip of the iceberg from inside. In apparently unrelated disease processes, eczema and asthma, sensitivities can manifest. Research also indicates that ingestion of aggressive food causes damage to the body over time, leading to several diseases and problems on the road.

Milk is such a normal allergy to a food that many people have been suffering for years because they don't accept that milk is an abuser. Or worse, people are frequently diagnosed as lactose intolerant and receive an extra lactase enzyme to never detect being responsive to other milk components such as whey or casesin. When lactose-only intolerance is involved, the additional form of lactase taken during dairy food also solves symptoms.

Blood checks may be carried out to test whether there is also real milk sensitivity. Some opt first for the elimination diet before beginning blood work only because it is "right now" possible without needles or doctors. Blood tests often allow for false positives, and the only way to be 100% positive if a milk sensitivity is reached is by removing all dairy products for a long time to see if the symptoms of sensitivity decrease. If they do, there is indeed a sensitivity, but some blood work may tell. If the symptoms disappear after milk is gone from the diet, the suspicion can also be easily checked by reintroducing milk to detect the symptoms coming back.

How and Why the No Flour-No Sugar Diet Works

No flour, no sugar = less calories

The trick to losing weight is literally to eat more calories than you do. My No Flour, No Sugar Diet works in the simplest sense because it lowers the calories to remove meal and extra sugar from your diet without altering other items. I discovered and checked the success of my patients that removing flour and sugar from your diet is an easy way to minimize calories quickly. For example, replacing high-calorie pieces of bread with low-calorie vegetables and legumes takes a lot of the calories without leaving you hungry or unmet. You can also feed your sweet tooth as you cut the calories by replacing sugar and honey with non-calorie sweeteners.

Compare the caloric content of two breakfasts — one with meal and sugar and one without, to see how the elimination of flour and sugar from your diet will significantly reduce the amount of calories you are consuming. When you usually start your day with bagels (ca. 250 calories), butter and strawberry jam (50 calories), and two teaspoons (30 calories) of coffee, you consume some 380 calories. Switching to an old-fashioned oatmeal (100 calories) with 1 cup of skim milk (90 calories), 80 calories medium apple, and ten calories artificial sweetener coffee can save you 110 calories. You will also have your fat consumption reduced from 7.5 grams to 2 grams, your fiber increased from 1 gram to 7 grams, and 400 mg calcium added. And just eggs. And that's breakfast.

As the above comparison shows clearly, removing meal and sugar from your diet is easy to get rid of any excess calories from your meals. As an extra benefit, you can automatically reduce the amount of fat that you consume. For example, without bread and jelly, what fun is high-fat peanut butter? No dinner, no cheesy pie, no cream-sauce pasta, and no buttery cookies. Remove sugar means no longer fat-filled ice cream or cake with frosting butter.

One pound of that fat is 3,500 calories. To lose one pound one week, you must eat 500 fewer calories a day or burn 500 more a day – or in a perfect world, a small part of either one. If, as in the breakfast example above, you could make dietary adjustments by taking off 110 calories from any meal that you consume, you'd easily be there more than halfway.

Stop meals of all sorts, including wheat, rice, and maize meals, or processed or condensed sugars (beet sugar, cane sugar, sucrose, glucose, molasses, honey, maple syrup, high fructose corn syrup, etc.). You can add bulk to your meals in the whole grains and stuffed vegetables, including wheat berries, barley, brown rice, maize, and potatoes. Enjoy fruit and fruit-sweetened goods to your sweet tooth - as long as they do not contain extra sugar. You can also taste sugar-free soda, gum, and even many of the now available light ice creams sweetened with Splenda or other artificial sweeteners. Snack on fresh fruit and raw vegetables – excellent low-calorie sources of major nutrients and fiber.

Cutting off your food's needless or "empty" calories is an easy and relatively painful way to achieve your aim. Further half an hour physical exercise a day – a short stroll, a tennis game, or a treadmill spin – you can easily expect to lose a pound a week before you hit your target weight.

Slow and steady wins the race.

While calorie reduction is necessary for weight loss, it is important to note that calories are the fuel of our bodies. They provide the energy we need to carry out normal daily work. While more calories than our bodies need can contribute to weight gain, even when you are trying to lose excess pounds, it is important to consume enough calories to receive the nutrients and energy that your body needs. Therefore, dietary and health professionals usually agree that certain diets that you lose no more than 1 or 2 pounds a week are the most successful.

To help you lose weight rapidly and drastically, many fad diets require a reduction in your caloric intake to levels insufficient to ensure that you get the nutrients you need. Moreover, when you avoid starving your body, the weight that is lost quickly is likely to return just as quickly. A gradual and steady approach will protect your health and deliver the results you want — and hold your weight off over time. Here and there, you're going to have a rough week, but don't be discouraged. It is the best of us. Even if you don't hit your one-pound goal within a given week, stick to the diet and the average weight loss over time.

A diet for (just about) everyone

Because my no flour, no sucrose diet, is ideal for almost everyone no matter what their age or level of activity, it promotes consuming several different types of foods from all food classes, including large quantities of nutrient-rich fruits, vegetables, and whole grains. All may benefit from taking empty calories from highly processed foods out of their diet, from young children to older people. People with serious medical problems — like diabetes, cardiac disease, high cholesterol, high blood pressure, etc. — are recommended to seek guidance from the medical doctor who treat them before making a substantial change in diet or activity level. In other words, No Flour, No Sugar Diet offers recommendations for balanced food that can be tailored to a wide variety of nutritional or medical needs.

Elimination Diets: The Gold Standard for Food Sensitivities?

Have you ever encountered the magnitude of a deprivation diet to see if foods in your diet cause uncomfortable symptoms? Most of us thought about it or at least thought about it. The classic disposal diet is now the gold standard for food sensitivities. To this day, we still use his definition. Many health care professionals, including medical physicians, regularly prescribe these diets.

And what exactly does an Elimination Diet entail? As it is well known, this type of diet attempts to remove for a period of time, usually 3 to 4 weeks, many of the common allergens (or as they should be named more accurately sensitivities) from the diet. This given the immune system plenty of time to calm down to see symptoms decrease. When food is reintroduced, the signs it produces are noticeable and more serious than before. This enables the recognition of the guilty foods.

Here are the foods typically eliminated on a basic elimination diet:

- Gluten
- Wheat
- Soy
- Corn
- Nightshades
- Dairy
- Peanuts
- Eggs

- Caffeine
- Alcohol
- Artificial Sweeteners
- Cane Sugar

Other foods eliminated on the stricter plans:
- Beans, lentils, peas
- ALL sugar (including honey, maple syrup, etc)
- All seeds and nuts
- Chicken
- Beef
- Shellfish
- Pork
- Certain chemicals (phenylethylamine, tyramine, MSG, nitrates, etc)

These diets, you might imagine, are obviously not a walk in the forest. They are usually recommended only for patients who are willing and willing to follow the protocol with the strong recommendation that a professional practitioner guides their diet. The rigor of the diet can be an obstacle for others, but proper knowledge, guidance, and encouragement can overcome this. Most of us dietitians have been educated and practiced during our training and are well prepared to go through the process.

Although you now know that there are elimination diets, you may have noticed that they have recently begun to become popular and almost boring in nature. There seem to be endless books on the shelves nowadays that speak about anti-inflammatory diet plans and advanced food plans that claim to help your weight loss, increase energy, and even make you look younger years. What are all these diets together? They are based on the classic diet!

As previously noted, these diets could be very restrictive or moderately restrictive, depending on the requirements. You and your doctor typically decide on this criterion and what foods they think are likely to be problematic in your unique situation. It is basically a guessing game, directed, educated, and well-meant. It's an even greater guessing match when you're following the strategy of some author who has never met you and doesn't know your past or symptoms.

And you've got the number one problem with our "gold standard." How did we decide what to cut and what to leave in the world? Why don't we advise someone to take apples or quinoa or other "healthy" foods that could be similarly troublesome, for example? If you are one of the few lucky ones who only respond to one or two popular allergens, this diet works very well for you. The problem has been solved! I met these people, and the diet for removal was a miracle. For others, it turned out to be yet another scheme that didn't succeed. Elimination diets can obviously be helpful, but not everyone's response. I know this firsthand because diets for removal never worked for me.

As I have already mentioned, several writers and experts are now advising various diets to cure your ailments and help you lose stubborn weight. Even Dr. Oz has a diet schedule for elimination! You know what you know now and can quickly check that this can be valid for a few. For many, these diets do not solve all the troublesome foods, and you have just spent money on another book or lost weeks of hard work for no benefit.

All this said I think the diets of elimination have their place. I had clients who were unable or reluctant to spend money on food allergy blood tests (the only thing I recommend is Oxford Biomedical Mediator Release Test), and we found a dietary plan that worked successfully for them. However, this is the minority. We've conjectured and won. That's not always the case. Many consumers who have already tried all appear to discover that no-one has noticed that they respond to random nutritious foods (i.e., vegetables, fruits, gluten-free grains, etc.) and have thus fallen through the cracks. Elimination diets demonstrate their drawbacks, and it is important to know the correct blood test to use.

The safest use of the elimination diet is with a certified physician who knows your whole health background and can help you prepare the best diet. The way to go is not a book, a TV show, or an online guide. Of course, these avenues have certainly helped some people, but the best alternative is a carefully adapted plan, particularly for people with more serious, chronic conditions. Naturally, blood testing is much more targeted if you find a doctor like me who provides mediator release testing. Train yourself on all the options before you start, or else all the hard work will be for nothing.

CHAPTER THREE

How to Lose Weight on the Low FODMAP Diet

How to Lose Weight on Low FODMAP Diet

It is not a diet that decreases weight, but certain weight fluctuation results from reducing or expanding their food choices. Most dietitians accept that successful loss of weight should not be carried out during the Low FODMAP Reduction and Challenge Process.

Why? Why? Both diets require attention to detail and prioritization of new diets and food choices. Trying to deal with both at the same time can be very difficult and can decrease the success rate for both purposes.

It is recommended highly to complete the low FODMAP elimination and FIRST challenge process in case you have a dual goal to monitor your IBS symptoms and weight loss.

A Dietitian Can Help

I have consulted with thousands of clients over the last two decades to seek weight loss through diet and exercise, loss of weight, and bariatric surgery. In the last four years, my focus has increased to include a FODMAP diet and IBS specialization.

Like all of us know, weight loss and weight management are difficult, very difficult. Nutrition science continues to advance in both areas, and a FODMAP trained RD will help you learn and help you to maximize this path.

Obesity remains a problem, considering the thousands of available diets and new weight loss drugs. Even radical methods like bariatric surgery do not prove foolish. The pendulum continues to change with different approaches to weight loss.

The guidelines for weight loss differ significantly, and sadly personal distortions set the tone for many. Dietitians teach evidence-based eating, often requiring practical and attainable lifestyle changes. The reality is that fad diets never equal long-term weight loss performance for weight reduction.

The low FODMAP diet is by no means a fad diet but is a scientific approach to reducing IBS symptoms. See our Licensed Dietitian Directory locate a dietitian near you.

What can you do, then?

These many tips that will help you lose weight after you've done the low FODMAP phases of elimination and challenge.

Watch your servings

Portion management in the low FODMAP diet is important since larger portions can reach healthy limits, rendering the food with low FODMAP FODMAP Food heavy. Minimizing the consumption of refined carbohydrates will enable you to slim down your waistline since they sometimes don't have a ton of fiber and contain unnecessary sugar.

Many foods are classified in grams or ounces in the low FODMAP Monash app and are therefore on a digital food level or even to measure cups and spoons will help raise awareness of acceptable and healthy serving sizes.

Eat at Regular Times

Try to eat three meals and 1 or 2 snacks throughout the day while you eliminate or minimize snacks late at night. Skip meals and eat large portions can lead to IBS symptoms and increase weight. Going without food for a long time can adversely affect the metabolic rate and also make us overeat and then make poor food choices – low FODMAP or not.

Burning most calories at night and eating at daytime is an all-too-usual trend of people struggling with their weight.

Miss breakfast and coffee fuel every morning are detrimental as both IBS and weight loss are handled. Try to spread the calories evenly during the day. Late-night snacks and huge dinners are a prescription for weight gain and sad tombs. Carry knowledge of why you snack – is hunger or habit connected? 1

Stay Hydrated

Every day, drink 64 to 80 ounces of water. Adequate hydration can help to lose weight and improve digestive health. Insufficient fluid and fiber may exacerbate IBS-C symptoms. Try to meet a measurable target to ensure that every day you exceed 64 to 80 ounces (2 L to 2.4 L).

For e.g., I fill up my hydro flask for 32 ounces (960 ml) twice a day, as well as additional drink fluids with food.

Sleep 7 to 8 Hours a Night

Chronic sleep deprivation tends to reduce the metabolic rate, increase portion preference, driving behaviors, increase the appetite hormone and decrease the hormone to make you feel whole.

Deprivation of sleep will fuel your cravings for unhealthy snacks and eat extra calories, sometimes more than 250 calories.

Bad sleep also tends to exacerbate IBS symptoms the next day, and IBS symptoms are more common for those reporting poor sleep quality. 2 There is also clear evidence that IBS individuals with increased sleep disorders versus healthy individuals are contributing to IBS development. 3

Eat More Plants

Try eating the rainbow and add color to your bowl. Make an effort to provide with every meal low FODMAP fruit and vegetables in safe portions.

Sometimes fiber consumption dips into a low FODMAP elimination diet, and hard work is done on the addition of plant-based fibres, including low FODMAP fruit and vegetables, canned and strained chickpeas and lentils, brown rice, oats, quinoa, candy, and winter squash (all in low FODMAP amounts, of course).

Fiber makes you breathe longer and monitors constipation. The low FODMAP diet also restricts the use of prebiotic fibres, which play an important role in intestinal health, and can reduce the negative impact of the ingestion of healthy portions of several plant-based fibers.

Don't Forget the Protein.

Often I feel like a pusher of protein. For starter protein, FODMAPs are not present, but they look for high FODMAP ingredients, such as garlic and onion, often combined with marinades and spices to taste the meat. None of us satisfy our needs for protein, but most of us eat protein at dinner and also with breakfast and lunch.

Adequate consumption of protein at each food will help mitigate the loss of lean muscle mass, which often accompanies the rapid loss of weight, marginally increases metabolic needs, and finally, helps you feel more complete. Four, fifth.

The healthy low protein choices for FODMAP include chicken, turkey, pork, shrimp, maize beef, pawns and chicken sausages (no garlic or onion), yogurt, lactose-free cottage cheese, and kefir, strained and consoled chickpeas, tofu, tempeh, and safe shakes or powders of protein.

Have a Plan

Meal preparation is the toughest aspect of any change in diet or new eating habits. We may all have good intentions, but if we do not have an action plan, the opportunity is significantly diminished to commit to new eating habits.

When blood sugar levels fall and time is limited, we sometimes reach a simple decision that is less likely to be safe and less likely to be low FODMAP. So what can we do... always try to prepare the next two dinners.

At breakfast you should think of dinner, maybe you should take out a portion of food for a last-minute item, or stop in the shop. Spend time for lunch, food, and preparing a few meals in advance.

Take short cuts such as purchasing precut fruit and vegetable tray or a small rotisserie chicken complying with FODMAP if time is tight.

Add Variety

I feel like many of us resort to our ancient ways when we are bored or caught in a rut. With your new eating habits, it is important to add new inspiration and exciting recipes. (Go to our FODMAP Everyday® Recipes page and use our filter to find what you want). Try not to get distracted by the overabundance of Internet recipes.

Try a new recipe or even a new spice once a week. This is more practical and would hopefully contribute to the rotation of new foods. Our recipes are various to try to check for our "kiwi" icon to see that Elimination Safe is a recipe.

Eat Fermented Foods

There is insufficient evidence to the support the use of weight loss probiotics. The weight gain was avoided despite substantially higher calories, and the strain Lactobacillus rhamnosus CGMCC1.3724 (LPR) in two small clinical trials showed that VSL #3 prevented weight gain in women.

Unfortunately, both the LPR probiotic supplement contained high FODMAP ingredients FOS and inulin. Both Align and VSL # 3 have shown their effectiveness in minimizing overall symptoms of IBS and improving the quality of life for more than eight weeks.

Consumption of these live crops can help to maintain stable Bifida levels that can be decreased in a low FODMAP diet. Six, seven, and eight. Low FODMAP probiotic food intake can increase the microbial diversity of gut bacteria, which can encourage a healthy weight.

Exercise

Take most days to work out. Find ways to move your body, whether it's walking, jogging, swimming, aerobics, yoga, or weight training. Most research indicates a target for safe weight loss and maintenance for 250 to 300 minutes a week.

Training can help alleviate stress, improve IBS, control IBS and improve digestion. Target moderate exercise since vigorous exercise may worsen IBS symptoms. 9

Be Mindful
We live in the society in which everything is done quickly, including food. Make attempts to eat food at a table without distractions like the TV, telephone, or reading.
Twenty times chew the food and try to eat slower. Deep breathing prior to a meal can help you remember to slow and alleviate stress, which can positively affect your IBS symptoms.

What Are High Fodmap Foods?

Will IBS and other diseases benefit from a low FODMAP diet?

- Low FODMAP diets are often used in numerous digestive problems, including IBS.
- These foods cause bowel syndrome irritable but can also exacerbate IBS symptoms. For IBS treatment, a low FODMAP diet is often recommended.
- •Functional GI disorders other than IBS
- •Small intestinal bacterial overgrowth (SIBO)

Experts believe that a diet plan that includes low FODMAPs can also help alleviate symptoms such as:

- Autoimmune diseases:
  - Eczema
  - Multiple sclerosis
  - Rheumatoid arthritis
- Fibromyalgia
- Migraines triggered by the certain eating products

After the diagnosis of your bowel disease or syndrome, e.g., IBS, IBD, or colitis, your doctor may suggest that your diet is low.

Symptoms and signs of too many high FODMAP foods
FODMAPs in the small intestine are not well absorbed. They increase the amount of fluid in the bowel and produce more gas.

Symptoms and signs suggesting that you can eat high in these short-chain carbohydrates are:

- Pain
- Gas
- Abdominal distention
- Bloating
- Diarrhea (similar to IBS symptoms)
- Abdominal pain
- A sense of fullness after a little food or liquid is eaten or drunk

A diet low in FODMAPs can help to alleviate these problems, especially in IBS individuals.

List of high FODMAP foods to avoid

Many foods that are high in FODMAPs otherwise constitute safe foods but can cause symptoms in some people with a sensitive intestine, particularly those with IBS or the other bowel diseases and the disorders like SIBO.

A list of popular foods to be avoided (especially if you have IBS) includes:

1. Some vegetables

- Garlic
- Onions
- Broccoli
- Cabbage
- Snow peas
- Cauliflower
- Artichokes
- Asparagus
- Beetroot
- Leeks

- Sweet corn
- Celery
- Mushrooms
- Brussels sprouts

2. Fruits, particularly "stone" fruits like:

- Apricots
- Peaches
- Plums
- Nectarines
- Mangoes
- Prunes
- Pears
- Apples
- Blackberries
- Cherries

3. Beans and lentils
4. Dried fruits and fruit juice concentrate
5. Wheat and rye

- Pizza
- Cereals
- Breads
- Crackers
- Pastas

6. Dairy products that contain lactose

- Soft cheese
- Milk

- Ice cream
- Yogurt
- Pudding
- Custard
- Cottage cheese

7. Nuts, including pistachios and cashews
8. Artificial sweeteners and Sweeteners

- Honey
- High fructose corn syrup
- Sorbitol
- Xylitol
- Agave nectar
- Maltitol
- Isomalt (commonly found in sugar-free gum and mints, and even cough syrups)
- Mannitol

9. Drinks

- Coconut water
- Sports drinks
- Alcohol

Fructose Malabsorption: Breaking It Down!

Malabsorption of Fructose (FM)

Fructose is a monosaccharide in three primary dietary forms:

1. A constitute of sucrose
2. Fructan
3. Free fructose

Fructose polymer, commonly in the form of the oligosaccharides, with terminal glucose considered to be also inulins, fructooligosaccharides (FOS), or oligofructose.

Fructose has become a monosaccharide (or simple sugar). Often known as fruit sugar is fructose. It is present in three major dietary forms: free fructose (in the case of honey or fruits), in the form of disaccharide sucrose, or in the form of fructus, a fructose polymer usually in the form of an oligosaccharide (present in wheat and some vegetables). This short chain of carbohydrates are commonly present in the diet as free fruit hexoses, as a sucrose disaccharide, and as fructus.

Fructose is found in many of the foods we consume, including natural and processed fruits and vegetables. Honey, agave syrup, fruit juices, pears, and apples are just some natural foods with substantial fructose ingredients. There is some fructose in all fruits, so portions are essential. Fructose is usually added in processed foods, beverages, and soft drinks as sulfur in the form of high fructose maize syrup.

Fructan is oligosaccharides and fructose-terminal polysaccharides. In many foods, these chains of fructose molecules are called fructans to occur naturally. Fructans alone produce gastrointestinal symptoms because the intestine is not hydrolyzed or absorbed. Fructans are a significant concern for patients with fructose malabsorption. Some high-fruit foods are maize, artichokes, leeks, onions, and inulin and fructooligosaccharides (FOS). Fiber is applied to some foods and supplements by inulin and fructooligosaccharide (FOS). If not entirely prevented, it is necessary to keep the amount of fructans in the diet small.

Glucose, also known as dextrose, is another monosaccharide, or plain sugar, in other words. Glucose is one of the simplest sugars to be used by most carbohydrates as a building block. Fructose and glucose also have almost the same caloric content, and fructose is a little sweeter. It is easier to digest fructose in combination with glucose. Also, with glucose intake, there is a limit on how well the body can absorb fructose. Glucose tablets are usually available in most medicines and food stores, usually in the diabetic or pharmaceutical section. For many recipes or sweeteners, dextrose powder (or glucose powder) may be used.

It is not as sweet as the sugar or fructose, but it is just sweet enough for many people. You can add more always. Some fruit products in recipes use a one-to-a-half ratio to replace glucose with sugar. Smarts and sweet-tart candies also have a big glucose component. These sweets can be consumed to digest excess fructose free. You must always check labels because here and there, they change their ingredients. Some have high fructose maize syrup, which is a big no-no to fructose sufferers. Glucose or dextrose should be the main ingredient. Labels are interpreted as being the primary ingredient, and in this order, the list continues with the last ingredient having the least number.

Two sugars are made of sucrose, fructose, and glucose. It is called double sugar consisting of one part of fructose and one part of glucose. Persons with fructose malabsorption can eat sucrose (limited quantities), as glucose helps with fructose absorption. Large quantities of sucrose can be problematic in one sitting as a large amount of fructose in all forms causes symptoms.

All human beings have limited fructose to absorb. The human intestine's ability to absorb fructose is limited and unique to every person. A healthy person can only consume 25 to 50 grams of fructose per session. Nobody has unlimited freedom to consume fructose, so that everyone has, to some extent, fructose malabsorption. Fructmal products are described as being capable of absorbing less than 25 grams per seat. The degree of malabsorption can vary from person to person.

Some people are very sensitive, and less fructose would possibly cause excess fructose to bloat and gas. As for lactose (a milk sugar contained in milk and milk products), people have a fructose threshold that can be ingested without causing symptoms. In fact, fructose malabsorption is written to be very normal, but it is unknown. Most citizens, including doctors and physicians, do not know what it is.

These days, high fructose maize syrup (HFCS) has received a lot of attention. High fructose maize syrup (HFCS) is a maize sweetener found in many foods and beverages in grocery shops in the USA. HFCS consists of either 42 or 55% fructose, while the remaining sugars are mainly glucose and higher sugars. There is the great deal of debate about how safe it is for consumption. Many claim it leads to obesity.

The Association of Corn Refiners claims that HFCS is natural and similar to table sugar. Research is underway to determine whether HFCS claims are true or incorrect. Sugar should be consumed in all forms in moderation for all. Elimination of HFCS is crucial if there is a desire to heal and live a healthy life for people who suffer from fructose malabsorption. Many processed foods and drinks are made from high-fructose maize syrup. The Corn Refiners Association is currently demanding that they change the name of the high fructose maize syrup into maize sugar.

People with fructose malabsorption must be mindful of four key aspects of their diets to prevent symptoms:
1. The total fructose in a meal
2. The fructose-glucose ratio in a meal
3. The existence of the polyols (sugar alcohols, like mannitol, xylitol, sorbitol, etc.)

4. The presence of the fructans (especially oligosaccharides, like FOS, Inulin, and short-chain di-, mono-, etc.)

IBS and SIBO: One and the Same?

Do you know any of these sounds? Painful bloating. Painful bloating. Irregular motions of the bowel (constipation, diarrhea, or both). Excess gas. Unnecessary gas. Tiredness. Flux. Flux. Abdominal cramping. Abdominal cramping. In other words, does your digestion suck in general?

For all of these forms of symptoms, Irritable Bowel syndrome is diagnosed (IBS). What is IBS? What is IBS? It affects the large intestine and triggers many of the symptoms mentioned above. In certain cases, it is a catch-all condition when other more established conditions have been ruled out, such as Crohn's or Ulcerative Colitis. IBS also does not cause intestinal harm, but it definitely causes a whole host of unpleasant symptoms. Treatment is usually dietary modifications and occasionally drugs to relieve the pain.

However, what we're finding of IBS now is that a substantial portion of people really doesn't have the big intestine as the only match. For others, the action actually happens in the small intestine (SI). Researchers have, in fact, discovered a condition by which bacterial imbalances occur in SI, which lays the stage for a whole host of symptoms similar to IBS. You name this small intestinal bacterial overgrowth (SIBO). Then what if... Just what if, really, all of these people "IBS" don't have IBS. What if this is SIBO?

Well, that's precisely what is reported. At present, it is estimated that some 20% of the population in this country is IBS, and about 60% is actually SIBO. That's definitely something to pause and remember. For several IBS patients, we concentrate on incorrect therapies.

So what is SIBO exactly, and how do we manage it? First, let's talk a bit about ordinary digestion so we can set the stage for SIBO's mistakes. Bear with me on this thrilling journey across the digestive tract.

When we chew and swallow, our acid arsenal is able to break down those amino acids and destroy unwanted bacteria that we eat. As food goes on its path through the system, it reaches the small intestine (SI), where the acid is neutralized, and digestive enzymes move in to split our meal and allow nutrient absorption. Any remaining material, particularly fiber and other undigested material, is forced into the colon and made ready for excretion. While I have greatly simplified this method, it's a very incredible operation.

Food instruction via the device is a peristalsis process call. We have peristalsis in the colon, and we force stools into the colon for excretion, and peristalsis in the small intestine, which moves food content to allow nutrient absorption and the rest to eventual excretion. At the SI, what we call the migrating motor complex, or the MMC, is coordinated by an important peristaltic motion. The MMC starts a cleansing wave in the fasting state, i. e. 90-120min after we eat that helps to push contents through and out of the IS. It also drives out the door unnecessary bacteria.

Furthermore, we have valves between each part of the digestive tract that help hold food where it should be and preferably travel downwards. We have the esophagus between the esophagus and the stomach and the ileoceal valve between the SI and the large intestine. Both are designed to stop backflow from the previous organ.

If all of the above works as intended, we have safe digestion. However, at any point of this delicate device, we may have malfunctioned and then set the stage for the SI to take hold of unwanted bacteria.

First, a person may lack sufficient stomach acid. Whilst this alone is not necessarily sufficient to cause SIBO, it can certainly aid, particularly in combination with other malfunctions. How many of us are on proton pump inhibitors in America? Or could H Pylori have? Low stomach acid is equivalent to poor digestion and a rise in SI bacteria.

There may also be a failure of the MMC feature inhibiting the washing wave that should eliminate the unwanted bacteria. This certainly leads to SIBO. What can lead to an MMC breakdown? Ok, for one, food poisoning. Food poisoning triggers a toxin that destroys the SI's nerves and prevents the MMC's operation. They are allowed to stay and set up shop instead of driving those requirements out. It can be a monumental job to get them out.

Another defect contributing to SIBO is ileocecal valve dysfunction. If the valve is defective and allows for large intestines to flow back, bacteria could reach the SI that should usually not be present. This once again sets the stage for the production of SIBO.

Structure abnormalities in the SI, which reduce movement of content and adhesions that allow bacteria to find a foothold and make a claim in the country of the SI, can also lead to other potential reasons. A convoluted mess like that, isn't it?

How do you understand if you have SIBO? Well, I find that a new onset of recurrent gas and extreme bloating is one sign. It's certainly not diagnostic, but it really reaches my ears. Diet also affects this, and consumers will remember that certain foods improve or make the condition worse.

The IBS-like symptoms that we mentioned earlier are other suggestions. In addition, a host of ambiguous symptoms can be linked initially to other causes. Reflux/GERD, tiredness, joint pain, headache/migraine, brain fog, and weight changes, etc. Any of these may be caused by SIBO food allergy reactions. SI bacteria raise the risk of leaky gut, as food sensitivity is also followed by SIBO. Malabsorption may also occur because of the bacteria damaging the SI brush border where our enzymes are formed. Less digestive enzymes are equivalent to less food absorption. Seriously, what an utter mess.

And what are we doing? Well, the first good move is to be checked. Yeah, tests are available to see if these buggers are in your system, thank you very much. If you do, you can use clear pharmaceutical and herbal protocols. These choices should be explored with a specialist MD or ND who can suggest the best course of action.

Dietary supplements can also be very effective and are an important part of the process. The truth is that some unwanted bacteria in the SI like to ferment carbohydrate substrates, so it can be useful in foods like FODMAPs, the special GAPs, carbohydrate diet, and others. I specialize in using these diets as a core part of SIBO management with customers.

Further lifestyle considerations may also help. These include spacing meals (let the MMC do that!), reduction of stress, and food safety (reduce the risk of food poisoning!). These are not only beneficial during recovery but also a crucial element in prevention.

In cases of digestive complaints, especially those with IBS, SIBO is clearly a critical consideration. Indeed, many IBS diagnoses disguise SIBO, as the symptoms frequently overlap between the two. It is to be hoped that SIBO awareness will continue to spread and will enable millions of people in this country to get the care required to cure a disease that is treatable but still not common in the gastrointestinal community.

A low-FODMAP diet is intended to help people with IBS manage their symptoms better by reducing certain foods. FODMAPs reflect oligo-saccharides, di-saccharides, mono-saccharides, and polyols that can be fermented. Simply put, FODMAPs are certain kinds of carbohydrates — sugars, starches, and food fiber.

Most of these things are not a concern if you don't consume them too much. Some people are susceptible to them, however.

FODMAPs draw water into your digestive tract that can bloat you. They will hang in your stomach and ferment if you eat too many of them.

CHAPTER FOUR

Laying a Foundation for a Healthy Life with Healthy Digestion

Our well-being affects our whole lives. It's our welfare. Building a wellness and well-being base is open the door to happiness. This is the base of our digestive system. What is ingested and how it is absorbed (or not absorbed) into our bodies affects us on a physical, mental and emotional level. Our internal cleaner is our digestive system. There is something that concerns our gastrointestinal health because it is very sensitive and fragile. In fact, something that does not damage the intestines is difficult to locate. It seems that they really get the low load of Everything. You won't be as lively and balanced as you could be when your g.i works without proper work. The method works best. To be at this top of the game, you must be careful to get along with your diet and Everything you consume. Food is your strength in survival. It is the greatest treatment, as nature serves all of us. Your GI is very critical and should never be underestimated. It takes great focus, just like Everything else that matters greatly in your life. A healthy digestive system results in ample energy, lightness in the body, sharp mental function, good eyesight, and balanced emotions, to name only a few.

Importance highlights

1. Really well, chew your food. The mechanical effect of chewing splits food into small parts, which are easier to strike with digestive juices. The chemical activities of salivary enzymes produced in the mouth by the salivary glands begin to digest carbohydrates.

2. Eat in a quiet and relaxing environment. Sit still and relax after a few minutes. Resting a few minutes after eating is a successful start to this very complex phase.

3. Eat raw fruit and not food between meals. For those with poor digestion, consuming raw fruit causes bowel gas and bloating with food. Cooked fruit could be more quickly digested as a dessert.

4. Eat meals freshly cooked. Try to stop as much as possible fast food and leftovers. Refrigerated foods are the most nutritious and free of mold or staleness.

5. Avoid overeating. Do not stuff yourself. Do not stuff yourself. Small foods are easier to digest and don't make you feel tired, heavy, and stuffed. Ancient Ayurvedic medicine recommends eating with two hands at every meal the sum of food that fits in two. Take time to leave the table and stop eating when you are still a little hungry. Moderate sections are more easily digested. Large foods put increased digestive demands as your body can produce only a certain amount of digestive juices.

6. Feed daily. Eat regularly. When you follow a daily routine, your digestive organs will function best. Even if you don't eat every meal or eat several meals, try to eat at the same amount.

7. Drink plenty of water every day but don't drink plenty of fluid at meals. Drinking too much during meals dilutes gastric juices and acids required to digest food. You have to remain hydrated, so drink between meals or restrict to one or two cups the amount you drink. There are some very critical organ systems that rely on water for your survival. If you don't drink enough water, your body takes the bowel with water, which is hard to move. Caffeine can also dehydrate as it acts as a diuretic, pushing water out of the body. Take note of chlorine and fluoride in your drinking water, among the other poor stuff. Drink reverse osmosis or pure water distilled. Add lemon slice and c vitamin to taste.

8. Defecate every day at the same time; even if you feel like you do not have to defecate, set a time to pass your intestines at the same time every day. The best time for breakfast is usually half an hour to an hour.

9. Get up and work. Get moving. Physical activity raises your breathing and heart rate and improves intestinal muscle activity, which helps to drive more food waste into your intestines faster. Exercise is an antidote to almost all that affects us. It boosts digestion and metabolism and all other physical, mental, and emotional health components.

10. Taking time to relax during your day, particularly when you eat, will not only improve your digestion but your health. Your emotions are both negative and optimistic, very strong. Get the feelings under control. Emotional upheavals and intense feelings can destroy your appetite, gut feeling, visceral reactions, give your stomach an upset, give you stomach butterflies or nervous intestines. Your stomach is a

muscle, and it can be very difficult to digest your food if you're up to or stressed out. This is because when your stomach is emotionally depressed or irritated, it is very difficult for you to digest a lot of anything. The battle or flight response you feel when you are stressed or threatened causes the body to respond by shutting down certain functions that are not required, like digestion, to run or fight. Many people are constantly fighting or traveling because of the unrelenting tension in our everyday lives. This puts a lot of pressure on digestion. Constant emotional upheaval doesn't allow your body time to regain calm, and your digestion can't do its job effectively. These emotions cause biochemical changes in your body when you are angry, stressed, or afraid. Various hormones and chemical compounds are released into your bloodstream.

Such negative thoughts stimulate the amygdala part of the brain. The amygdala is linked directly to the abdomen. Any emotion that affects your brain portion also affects your digestion. If you create toxic emotional responses by triggering your amygdala through fear, rage, or anxiety, these chemicals stay 72 hours-3 days in your bloodstream, even when neutralized. If the body fears, the grip induces dramatic changes that can directly impact digestion, leading to poor digestion and poor health. Chronic concern and stress is a cause for great pain, including colitis and irritable bowel syndrome. Emotionally disturbed, it is best not to feed. Blessed emotions affect physiological processes in the body, as well as negative emotions. If we're relaxed, carefree, and happy, we don't get them sick. Improved digestion is one consequence of a happy disposition. Take measures to restore equilibrium and release negative emotions, especially before you eat. Positive feelings can improve your digestion, improve your health, and sometimes even heal your pain. It neutralizes not only the effects of negative emotions on your digestion but also encourages a healthy heart. Your emotions and metabolism would not be able to recover without decompression.

Relaxation and lack of concern are highly necessary to ensure that the digestive process is at its peak. If you change your thoughts consciously from anger, fear, or anxiety to love and goodness, the change in brain chemistry dispels emotional toxins. When we feel good about our climate, we appreciate our food more and easily assimilate it. It makes eating a pleasure and digestion progress to be around us with good companionship, friendly conversation, and a safe setting. Walking after dinner and joking after dinner allows food to pass through the digestive tract more quickly. When we relax, our belly and other organs are less tense, less constrained, and more readily able to accomplish their tasks.

11. Limit sugar, salt, bleached and refined foods consumption. Small amounts won't affect you, but too many of these and the whole system have a significant effect.

12. Eat a fiber-resistant diet. Try adding fiber tablets or blends to your diet if you don't get enough fiber in foods. For a healthy digestive system, fiber is important. Many options are available. (If you have fructose malabsorption, you don't want Inulin or Fructo-oligosaccharides labeled with fiber (FOS). They are both added to foods and supplements to add more nutrition to the diet.)

13. Limit consumption of bad fats and fried foods like potato chips, cakes, and cookies. There are various types of fats. Any of them are excellent for you and vital for a balanced body, spirit, and digestive system. Extra virgin olive oil, avocados, salmon, and nutrients are some examples of healthy fat foods.

14. Hot water is a perfect way of detoxifying the body and building digestive muscle. Drink a glass of hot water with lemon in the morning

or drink it all day. It helps purify the digestive tract and blocks and impurities in the body. Drinking hot water increases digestion and food assimilation and helps prevent the body from being acidic and obstructive.

15. Try eating organic as much as you can. Many people are susceptible, allergic, and intolerant to our food chemicals.

16. Wear olive oil. The most digestible of the all edible fats is extra-virgin olive oil. It's great for your heart and has a very positive effect on digestion, prevention, and cure.

17. Stop heavy alcohol intake, which can result in digestive disturbances. Alcohol can also exacerbate symptoms, including diarrhea or nausea. It can also spark your stomach furnace and calm your lower esophagus.

18. Many medications on the counter and prescription, even in large amounts, impair digestion. Do your homework before you take some medicines. High blood pressure medicines, for example, can cause diarrhea or constipation. Non-steroidal inflammatory medicines (NSAIDs). Like aspirin, ibuprofen (Advil, Motrin, others), and naproxen (Aleve), if taken occasionally or above the administered dose, it can cause nausea, stomach pain, stomach bleeding, ulcers, or diarrhea. Narcotics can cause constipation and nausea. And some nausea or diarrhea can be caused by antibiotics.

19. Kick the habit of nicotine. Tobacco nicotine can increase the production of stomach acid and reduce the production of sodium bicarbonate, a substance that neutralizes the stomach acid. During smoking, air swallowed may cause belching or gas bloating. The risk of Crohn's disease is also predicted to increase with nicotine.

20. Food allergies and intolerances are numerous. The most popular food allergy is milk. These days, gluten and wheat are also common

villains. It is important to find a meal plan for you. You want to feed your body, not to poison it.

21. Celiac disease is a genetically induced autoimmune disease characterized by small intestinal mucosa recurrent inflammation. Persons with celiac conditions have an immunological response to certain amino acid sequences present in grains of wheat, rye, and barley. When anyone has celiac disease, they cause an immune system response that affects the small intestinal mucosa. Inflammation and vile atrophy can lead to nutrient malabsorption. Symptoms include diarrhea, stomach pain, cramping, and bloated abdominal distension ness, for example. The (chronic) pale, voluminous, and malodorous diarrhea characteristic of coeliac disease. A degree of lactose intolerance may develop as the bowel gets more damaged.

The signs are sometimes due to irritable bowel syndrome (IBS), later only as celiac disease. For those with IBS symptoms, celiac disease screening is recommended. The extreme celiac condition leads to pale, loose, and grassy stool symptoms and to weight loss or non-weight gain (in young children). People with milder celiac disease can have more subtle signs, which arise in other organs than in the intestines themselves. However, celiac disease is possible without any symptoms at all. Many adults suffering from subtle illness have only fatigue or anemia. As a result of increased screening, increasing portions of diagnoses are made in asymptomatic individuals. A small bowel biopsy is diagnosed for celiac disease.

Blood testing is useful for screening for coeliac diseases, including: Tissue Transglutaminase (IGA). Antigliadin Antibodies (IgA and IgG), Endomysia Antibodies (IgA), and Complete IgA. You should be screened for coeliac disease if you are suspected you may or might have the disease. If you have a celiac disorder, long-term gluten intake can be very harmful, so information is important. The long-term and untreated celiac disease might lead to complications, including ulceration of the small bowel and narrowing due to bowel blockage.

Untreated celiac disease also raises the risk of small bowel cancer and bowel lymphoma. Proper diet therapy will help to minimize these risks. It is very important to be screened correctly for coeliac disease prior to gluten removal; otherwise, a positive or negative diagnosis cannot be easily obtained. However, you should have a gene test done if you're on a gluten-free diet already.

22. Keep away from olestra-containing goods. It is primarily an ingredient in chips. It is a synthetic fat replacement that is not consumed by the human body but causes two issues. It can cause gastrointestinal problems, especially in some people, abdominal clamping and loose stools. The absorption of certain vitamins and the other nutrients may be impaired.

23. Keep yourself aspartame safe. Aspartame, which is publicly referred to as NutraSweet, Equal, and Spoonful, is known to cause all kinds of digestive distress, including stomach cramps and diarrhea. Aspartame isn't good for you in the end. Let's start simple. Just start simple. It does not have a nutritional value. Aspartame is foreign, alien, and causes multiple lists of side effects, unlike sugar that your body needs. Headache, epileptic seizures known as tiny malfunctions, and several other unpleasant side effects have been recorded.

24. Tap water includes many of the toxins that are digestive and health agents, including chlorine and fluoride. The value of the purest possible water cannot be emphasized enough.

25. Food poisoning can vary between mild and serious. Left-over in the refrigerator can cause milder forms of food poisoning. Bacteria collect on the left surface that the human eye cannot see. Follow the rule of three days and throw out any remains on the third day.

Straightforward Tips for A Diabetic Diet Program and Eating Sensibly

It is important to eat properly in accordance with your diabetic diet program. A big part of life with diabetes is the consumption of healthy, wholesome foods and healthier life. Changing your style of life is important as a diabetic person; a change of lifestyle will avoid cardiovascular problems that could destroy you right if you are left ignored.

If you consume unhealthy foods in the past and you have become unwanted in weight, various eating plans have come about to fix this particular unhealthy issue.

Consume more food and weight sheds - A lot of small food is the key ingredient to accelerate your metabolism. Sweets and most foods with heavily refined sugars must be totally abandoned, as they greatly raise blood sugar levels.

Eating less calories than your real body mass index will slow down your metabolic process and result in weight gain rather than weight loss. Experience decreasing and increasing your calories and calories by exercising before you find a technique that works for you.

Most people equate weight loss with being boring and hungry, but they can eat better while still losing unwelcome excess pounds. A balanced, low-calorie diet could make you feel much more energy satisfied. It allows long overdue employment to be tackled or a brand-new hobby pursued. Consume mostly real foods - meats, fish, dairy, fat milk products, salads, fresh vegetables, fresh fruits, and whole grain.

Eat fat reduced nutritious foods - This is extremely simple because of the low-fat options in supermarkets and health food stores. Eat six or five small meals a day, such as a ton of nutritious carbohydrates, to keep you alert and happy, along with uninterrupted amounts of glucose, throughout the day. Excess weight around your stomach poses an increased overall health risk – adopt a balanced eating plan to get the perfect shape.

Using a normal amount of food per day and prescription medications will boost blood glucose control dramatically and minimize the chances of diabetes-related hazards, such as coronary artery disease, renal health issues, and nerve impairment. Furthermore, feeding frequently affects your weight management.

Learn natural proteins can also be very important, especially proteins that are an excellent source of essential omega-three fatty acids in a variety of seafood such as salmon.

Exercise - this is really encouraged for people who try to lose weight but is also particularly beneficial for people with diabetes. However, like anything new, to make sure that you don't overdo it, it is really important to track blood sugar levels before and after exercise. Early morning workouts will eat more calories out of the fat.

Training has many health and wellness benefits - Strengthening training exercises like those on physical fitness equipment helps protect the bones and make vital joints more flexible. Exercise every day at the same time. This will help encourage a more stable level of blood sugar.

Exercise helps you throw away pounds by developing muscle tissue and eating fat calories. This can take time, of course, particularly to spot the differences; each individual activity becomes much easier and healthier. It is important to do daily exercises to ensure that you have a good fitness level.

Physical exercise can turn fat into denser, heavier muscle tissue that maintains body weight identical while improving heart and wellness all over the world. Add to daily workouts an outstanding balanced diet.

In reality, type 1 diabetes is a lifelong condition without cure (so far), but the outlook on life for people battling this disease is far exceeded 20 years ago. Numerous breakthroughs have occurred in medication, testing, and awareness, reducing any weakening issues and increasing life expectancy for people without type 1 diabetes at a stage.

Diabetes type one is much less common than diabetes type 2 and may not affect younger people. It is primarily seen in men and women less than 40 years of age and in children less than 14 years of age.

However, type 2 diabetes develops very slowly without any signs or symptoms. Regrettably, type 2 diabetes is only commonly known after a condition arises, for example, blood circulation disorders, nerve damage, vision impairment, or damage to the renal system. Type 2 diabetes is treated through diet and physical activity, tablet or insulin alone, or by physical activity.

Choosing a beneficial diabetic weight loss diet is as simple as choosing which delicious foods you would definitely enjoy. The timing of daily meals is an important aspect of a diet regimen for diabetics.

Safe and nutritious food choices are important for all, but their value cannot be over-determined for a particular type 2 diabetes patient. Regulation of blood glucose levels is important to avoid numerous diabetes problems. Diabetic health agencies must serve as advocates for patients and ask them to discuss their specific diseases with other diabetic patients.

Researchers also found that excess fat around your stomach leads to a much higher risk of health issues like cardiovascular disease and certain types of cancer. You find that if the majority of your excess fat is inside the stomach region, your health issues may be more serious relative to other areas of the body. However, the research is contradictory whether it is solely due to menopause or to an age group entirely (just because males are as weighty as they grow old), or even a combination of age and menopause.

Health practitioners help weight loss patients to control their diabetic problems. Adjusting food habits and weight loss can be difficult for some people with this condition. Medical practitioners have the means to assess the effect of a certain carbohydrate food on a person's level of blood sugar. This is known as the index list of glycaemics.

Health professionals want their patients to get a good bodyweight just like the patient, so it's crucial that you interact to achieve this. If weight loss goals advance, several appointments with your healthcare provider might be appropriate.

Dietary fiber is very important for a diabetes patient because soluble fiber influences blood glucose levels. Dietary fiber food products are not only suitable for colon cleaning but also benefit from a weight loss program.

Carbohydrate foods also referred to as carbohydrates, provide vitality with glucose. High-fiber foods, apples, milk, vegetables like maize, and sugar are all carbohydrate foods. Carbohydrates are usually transformed very early in digestive activity into all kinds of sugar. It is important to get a refresher course from your dietician on carbohydrates and how to measure them.

Carbohydrates that have very little nutritional advantage, such as sweet sugar, white bread, and other products made with white meal, must be ruled out. Keep an easy meal plan that includes uncomplicated, sweet foods and delicious recipes that can help you regulate blood sugar. Your body converts superior carbohydrates into glucose, providing your body with energy.

Very large quantities of poor carbohydrate intake generate higher levels of blood glucose, significantly impacting diabetic patients. The lack of desire to avoid eating characterizes carbohydrate craving. You probably want strong snacks all day long, and sweets right after you eat. The introduction during the day of snack foods with reduced carbohydrates (banana, apple, or any negative food) could help fill your stomach's emptiness.

A healthy snack is often small chicken or turkey bits, and snacking every 3 hours of the day is a great help in maintaining your level of glucose.

Try a FODMAPs diet to manage irritable bowel syndrome

Irritable bowel syndrome (IBS) is the common gastrointestinal disorder in the United States, affecting one out of 10 people every year. It is no surprise which living with IBS can have a significant impact on a person's quality of life with symptoms like cramping, diarrhea, gas, and bloating.

Diet is one way to manage symptoms of IBS. A common approach to treatment is to avoid foods that cause symptoms. Another IBS diet, developed in Australia, is very successful in IBS symptoms management. It is referred to as the low FODMAP diet.

Researchers have found that the small intestine is not well able to absorb FODMAPs. They increase fluid content in the bowel and also generate more gas. It is because colonic bacteria ferment easily in the colon. Increased fluid and gas in the bowel can result in bloating and speed changes with which food is digested.

Studies have shown that low FODMAP diets improve IBS symptoms, and one study has even found that 76 percent of IBS patients have improved their symptoms following the diet.

EAT LESS OF THESE FOODS
• Lactose
  • Cow's milk, pudding, yogurt, ice cream, custard, mascarpone, cottage cheese,

• Fructose
  • Fruits such as pears, apples, cherries, peaches, pears, mangoes, and watermelon

- Sweeteners, such as agave nectar and honey
- High fructose maize syrup products

• Fruitans
- Vegetables such as asparagus, artichokes, broccoli, Brussels sprouts, garlic, beetroot, and onions
- Grains like rye and wheat
- Added fiber, for example, inulin.

• GOS.
- Lentils, Chickpeas, soy products, and kidney beans
- Vegetables, such as broccoli

• Polyols.
- Fruit such as apricots, apples, cherries, blackberries, pears, nectarines, plums, peaches, and watermelon
- Vegetables such as cauliflower, snow peas and mushrooms
- Sweeteners such as sorbitol, mannitol, xylitol, isomalt and maltitol found in gum and mints free of sugar, cough and drops.

Eat more of the food.
- Dairy: rice milk, lactose-free milk, coconut milk, almond milk, lactose-free yogurt.
- Fruit: strawberries, bananas, cantaloupe, blueberries, honeydew, grapefruit, lemon, kiwi, oranges, and lime, and
- Vegetables: bean sprouts, Bamboo shoots, carrots, bok choy, cucumbers, chives, ginger, eggplant, olives, lettuce, potatoes, parsnips, turnips, and spring onions.

- Protein: pork, Beef, fish, chicken, tofu, and eggs
- Nuts/seeds (limited by 10 to 15): macadamia, almonds, pine nuts, peanuts, and walnuts.
- Grain: oat bran, oat, rice bran, gluten-free pasta like maize, rice, white rice, quinoa, maize, and quinoa.

The idea behind a low FODMAP diet is to limit only problem foods within one category – not all of them. (They have health benefits after all.)

If you're considering this diet, meet with a registered dietician. It's important that you make sure your diet is healthy and safe. He or she will have you take away the FODMAP from your diet. Then you gradually add carbs one at a time and monitor your symptoms.

Some healthcare professionals think the low FODMAP diet is too restrictive. Diet proponents report that people stick to it because of how it improves their quality of life.

CHAPTER FIVE
Fodmap Foods

High FODMAP food (things to avoid / reduce)

Vegetables and Legumes

Garlic – Includes garlic powder, garlic salt

- Onions – avoid
  - Includes small pickled onions, onion powder,

Try Hing / garlic oil or Asafoetida powder to substitute

- Asparagus
- Artichoke
- Beetroot, fresh
- Baked beans
- Broad beans
- Black eyed peas
- Cassava
- Butter beans
- Celery – greater than 5cm of stalk
- Cauliflower
- Falafel
- Choko
- Haricot beans
- Fermented cabbage e.g. sauerkraut
- Lima beans
- Kidney beans
- Mange Tout

- Leek bulb
- Mung beans
- Mixed vegetables
- Peas, sugar snap
- Mushrooms
- Red kidney beans
- Pickled vegetables
- Soy beans / soya beans
- Savoy Cabbage – over 1/2 cup
- Scallions / spring onions (bulb / white part)
- Split peas
- Taro
- Shallots

Fruit – fruits could contain high fructose

- Apples including pink lady and granny smith
- Avocado
- Apricots
- Blackberries
- Bananas, ripe
- Boysenberry
- Blackcurrants
- Currants
- Cherries
- Dates
- Custard apple
- Figs
- Feijoa
- Grapefruit – over 80g
- Goji berries
- Lychee

- ➢ Guava, unripe
- ➢ Nectarines
- ➢ Mango
- ➢ Peaches
- ➢ Paw paw, dried
- ➢ Persimmon
- ➢ Pears
- ➢ Plums
- ➢ Pineapple, dried
- ➢ Prunes
- ➢ Pomegranate
- ➢ Sea buckthorns
- ➢ Raisins – over 1 tbsp / 13g
- ➢ Tamarillo
- ➢ Sultanas
- ➢ Watermelon
- ➢ Tinned fruit in pear juice / apple

Poultry, Meats, and Meat Substitutes
- Sausages
- Chorizo if garlic added

Cereals, Breads, Grains, Cookies/ Biscuits, Nuts, Pasta, and Cakes
- ➢ Wheat containing products such as (be sure to check labels):
- o Bread, wheat – over 1 slice
- o Biscuits / cookies including chocolate chip cookies
- o Cakes
- o Breadcrumbs
- o Croissants
- o Cereal bar, wheat based

- Egg noodles
- Crumpets
- Pastries
- Muffins
- Udon noodles
- Pasta, wheat over 1/2 cup cooked
- Wheat cereals
- Wheat bran
- Wheat germ
- Wheat flour
- Wheat rolls
- Wheat noodles

- Amaranth flour
- Almond meal
- Bran cereals
- Barley including flour

- Bread:
  - Multigrain bread
  - Sourdough with kamut
  - Granary bread
  - Oatmeal bread
  - Naan
  - Roti
  - Pumpernickel bread

- Chestnut flour
- Cashews
- Einkorn flour
- Cous cous

- ➢ Gnocchi
- ➢ Freekeh
- ➢ Muesli cereal
- ➢ Granola bar
- ➢ Pistachios
- ➢ Muesli bar
- ➢ Rye crispbread
- ➢ Rye
- ➢ Spelt flour
- ➢ Semolina

Dips, Condiments, Sweeteners, Sweets, and Spreads

- ➢ Caviar dip
- ➢ Agave
- ➢ Fruit bar
- ➢ Fructose
- ➢ High fructose corn syrup (HFCS)
- ➢ Gravy, if it contains onion
- ➢ Honey
- ➢ Hummus / houmous
- ➢ Jam, strawberry, if contains HFCS
- ➢ Jam, mixed berries
- ➢ Pesto sauce
- ➢ Molasses
- ➢ Relish / vegetable pickle
- ➢ Quince paste
- ➢ Stock cubes
- ➢ Sugar free sweets containing polyols – usually ending in -ol or isomalt
- ➢ Sweeteners and corresponding E number:
- o Isomalt (E953 / 953)
- o Xylitol (E967 / 967)

- o Inulin
- o Maltitol (E965 / 965)
- o Lactitol (E966 / 966)
- o Sorbitol (E420 / 420)
- o Mannitol (E241 / 421)

- ➤ Tzatziki dip

Prebiotic Foods
- o The follow items might be hiding in snack bars, yoghurts, etc:
- o Oligofructose
- o Inulin
- o FOS – fructooligosaccharides

Drinks and Protein Powders
- ➤ Cordial, apple and raspberry with 50-100% real juice
- ➤ Beer – if drinking more than one bottle
- ➤ Fruit and herbal teas with apple added
- ➤ Cordial, orange with 25-50% real juice
- ➤ Fruit juices made of apple, pear, mango
- ➤ Fruit juices in large quantities
- ➤ Malted chocolate flavored drink
- ➤ Kombucha
- ➤ Orange juice in quantities over 100ml
- ➤ Meal replacement drinks containing milk-based products e.g. Ensure, Slim Fast
- ➤ Rum
- ➤ Quinoa milk
- ➤ Soymilk made with soy beans – commonly found in USA

- ➢ Sodas containing High Fructose Corn Syrup (HFCS)
- ➢ Sports drinks

- ➢ Tea:
- o Chai tea, strong
- o Black tea with added soymilk
- o Fennel tea
- o Dandelion tea, strong
- o Herbal tea, strong
- o Chamomile tea
- o Oolong tea
- o Wine – if drinking more than one glass

- ➢ Whey protein, hydrolyzed unless lactose free
- ➢ Whey protein, concentrate unless lactose free

Dairy Foods
- ➢ Cheese, ricotta
- ➢ Kefir
- ➢ Buttermilk
- ➢ Custard
- ➢ Cream
- ➢ Ice cream
- ➢ Gelato

- ➢ Milk:
- o Goat milk
- o Cow milk
- o Sheep's milk

- o Evaporated milk

- ➤ Yoghurt
- ➤ Sour cream – over 2tbsp

Cooking ingredients
Carob flour / Carob powder

Low FODMAP food (good to eat food)

If quantities are given these are the highest amount allowed

A great source of ready made and flavorful low FODMAP sauces, oils and snacks is FODY Foods.

Vegetables and Legumes

Bamboo shoots
- ➤ Alfalfa
- ➤ Beetroot, canned and pickled
- ➤ Bean sprouts
- ➤ Bok choy / pak choi
- ➤ Black beans – 1/4 cup / 45g
- ➤ Broccoli, heads only – 3/4 cup
- ➤ Broccoli, whole – 3/4 cup
- ➤ Broccolini, whole – 1/2 cup chopped
- ➤ Broccoli, stalks only – 1/3 cup
- ➤ Broccolini, stalks only – 1 cup
- ➤ Broccolini, heads only – 1/2 cup
- ➤ Butternut squash – 1/4 cup
- ➤ Brussels sprouts – 2 sprouts
- ➤ Callaloo
- ➤ Cabbage, common and red up to 3/4 cup
- ➤ Celeriac
- ➤ Carrots

- ➢ Chicory leaves
- ➢ Celery – less than 5cm of stalk
- ➢ Chilli – if tolerable
- ➢ Chick peas – 1/4 cup
- ➢ Cho cho – 1/2 cup diced
- ➢ Chives
- ➢ Collard greens
- ➢ Choy sum
- ➢ Courgette – 65g
- ➢ Corn / sweet corn
- ➢ Eggplant / aubergine (1 cup)
- ➢ Cucumber
- ➢ Green beans
- ➢ Fennel
- ➢ Ginger
- ➢ Green pepper / green bell pepper / green capsicum – 1/2 cup
- ➢ Karela
- ➢ Kale
- ➢ Lentils – in small amounts
- ➢ Leek leaves

Lettuce:
- o Iceberg lettuce
- o Butter lettuce
- o Red coral lettuce
- o Radicchio lettuce
- o Romaine/Cos lettuce
- o Rocket lettuce

- ➢ Okra
- ➢ Marrow
- ➢ Parsnip

- Olives
- Pickled gherkins
- Peas, snow – 5 pods
- Potato
- Pickled onions, large
- Pumpkin, canned – 1/4 cup, 2.2 oz
- Pumpkin
- Red capsicum / red bell pepper / Red peppers
- Radish
- Seaweed / nori
- Scallions / spring onions (green part)
- Spaghetti squash
- Silverbeet / chard
- Squash
- Spinach, baby
- Swede
- Sun-dried tomatoes – 4 pieces
- Sweet potato – 1/2 cup
- Swiss chard
- Tomato –cherry, canned, roma, common
- Tomato, canned – 3/5 cup
- Tomato, cherry – 5 cherries
- Tomato, common – 1 small
- Tomatillos, canned – 75g
- Tomatillo, fresh – 1 cup
- Water chestnuts
- Turnip – 1/2 turnip
- Zucchini – 65g
- Yam

Fruit

- Bananas, unripe – 1 medium
- Ackee
- Blueberries – 1/4 cup
- Bilberries
- Carambola
- Breadfruit
- Cranberry – 1 tbsp
- Cantaloupe – 3/4 cup
- Coconut, cream – 1/4 cup
- Clementine
- Dragon fruit
- Coconut, flesh – 2/3 cup
- Grapes
- Lingonberries
- Honeydew and Galia melons – 1/2 cup
- Guava, ripe
- Lemon including lemon juice
- Kiwifruit – 2 small
- Mandarin
- Lime including lime juice
- Passion fruit
- Orange
- Papaya
- Paw paw
- Plantain, peeled
- Pineapple
- Raspberry – 30 berries
- Prickly pear / nopales
- Strawberry
- Rhubarb
- Tangelo
- Tamarind

Poultry, Meats, and Meat Substitutes

- Chicken
- Beef
- Foie gras
- Chorizo
- Lamb
- Kangaroo
- Prosciutto
- Pork
- Turkey
- Quorn, mince
- Processed meat – check ingredients
- Cold cuts / deli meat / cold meats such as ham and turkey breast

Fish and Seafood

- Canned tuna
- Fresh fish e.g.
  - Haddock
  - Cod
  - Salmon
  - Plaice
  - Tuna
  - Trout

- Seafood (ensuring nothing else is added) e.g.
  - Lobster
  - Crab
  - Oysters

- o Mussels
- o Shrimp
- o Prawns

Grains, Cereals, Biscuits, Breads, Nuts, Pasta, and Cakes

- ➢ Wheat free breads
- ➢ Gluten free breads
- ➢ Bread:
- o Rice bread
- o Corn bread
- o Potato flour bread
- o Spelt sourdough bread

- ➢ Bread, wheat – 1 slice
- ➢ Wheat free or gluten free pasta
- ➢ Biscuit, cream cracker – 4 crackers
- ➢ Almonds – 10 almonds
- ➢ Biscuit, savory – 2 biscuits
- ➢ Biscuit, oatcakes – 4 cakes
- ➢ Biscuit, sweet, plain – 2 biscuits
- ➢ Biscuit, shortbread – 1 biscuit
- ➢ Brazil nuts
- ➢ Biscuit, wholegrain oat cereal biscuit – 2 biscuits
- ➢ Buckwheat
- ➢ Bulgur / bourghal – 1/4 cup cooked, 44g serving
- ➢ Buckwheat noodles
- ➢ Buckwheat flour
- ➢ Chestnuts
- ➢ Brown rice / whole grain rice
- ➢ Cornflour / maize
- ➢ Chips, plain / potato crisps, plain

- Corncakes
- Crispbread
- Cornflakes, gluten free
- Cornflakes – 1/2 cup
- Corn tortillas, 3 tortillas
- Corn, creamed and canned (up to 1/3 cup)
- Flax seeds / linseeds – up to 1 tbsp
- Crackers, plain
- Hazelnuts – 10 hazelnuts
- Kellogg's (US):
  - Crispix
  - Corn Flakes
  - Rice Krispies
  - Frosted Krispies
  - Frosted Flakes

- Millet
- Macadamia nuts
- Oatmeal, 1/2 cup
- Mixed nuts
- Oatcakes
- Oats
- Pecans – 10 halves
- Peanuts
- Polenta
- Pine nuts
- Porridge and oat based cereals
- Popcorn
- Pretzels
- Potato flour
- Pasta, wheat – up to 1/2 cup cooked

- ➢ Quinoa
- ➢ Rice: (Brown rice, Basmati rice, White rice, Rice noodles, Rice flour)
- ➢ Rice cakes
- ➢ Rice bran
- ➢ Rice flakes
- ➢ Rice crackers
- ➢ Seeds: (Dill seeds, Chia seeds, Hemp seeds, Egusi seeds, Pumpkin seeds, Poppy seeds, Sesame seeds)
- ➢ Starch, maize, potato and tapioca
- ➢ Sunflower seeds
- ➢ Tortilla chips / corn chips
- ➢ Sorghum
- ➢ Walnuts

Condiments, Dips, Sweets, Sweeteners and Spreads

- ➢ Acesulfame K
- ➢ Aspartame
- ➢ Barbecue sauce – check label carefully
- ➢ Almond butter
- ➢ Capers, salted
- ➢ Capers in vinegar
- ➢ Chocolate: (White chocolate – 3 squares, Milk chocolate – 4 squares, Dark chocolate – 5 squares)
- ➢ Dijon mustard
- ➢ Chutney, 1 tablespoon
- ➢ Fish sauce
- ➢ Erythritol (E968 / 968)
- ➢ Glucose
- ➢ Golden syrup – 1 tsp
- ➢ Jam / jelly, strawberry

- Glycerol (E422 / 422)
- Ketchup (USA) – 1 sachet
- Jam / jelly, raspberry – 2 tbsp
- Marmalade
- Maple syrup
- Mayonnaise – ensuring no garlic or onion in ingredients
- Marmite
- Mustard
- Miso paste
- Pesto sauce – less than 1 tbsp
- Oyster sauce
- Rice malt syrup
- Peanut butter
- Shrimp paste
- Saccharine
- Sriracha hot chilli sauce – 1 tsp
- Soy sauce
- Sweet and sour sauce
- Stevia
- Sugar – also called sucrose
- Sucralose
- Tamarind paste
- Tahini paste
- Vegemite
- Tomato sauce (outside USA) – 2 sachets, 13g
- Vinegars: (Rice wine vinegar, Balsamic vinegar, 2 tbsp, Apple cider vinegar, 2 tbsp)
- Worcestershire sauce – has onion and garlic but very very low amount making it low FODMAP
- Wasabi

Drinks and Protein Powders

- ➤ Alcohol – is an irritant to the gut, limited intake advised: (Clear spirits such as Vodka, Wine – limited to one drink, Whiskey Beer – limited to one drink, Gin)
- ➤ Coffee:
- o Espresso coffee, regular or decaffeinated, with up to 250ml lactose free milk
- o Instant coffee, regular or decaffeinated, with up to 250ml lactose free milk
- o Espresso coffee, regular or decaffeinated, black
- o Instant coffee, regular or decaffeinated, black

- ➤ Coconut, water – 100ml
- ➤ Coconut, milk – 125ml
- ➤ Fruit juice, 125ml and safe fruits only
- ➤ Drinking chocolate powder
- ➤ Lemonade – in low quantities
- ➤ Kvass
- ➤ Protein powders:
- o Pea protein – up to 20g
- o Egg protein
- o Whey protein isolate
- o Sacha Inchi protein
- o Rice protein

- ➤ Soya milk made with soy protein
- ➤ Tea:
- o Chai tea, weak
- o Black tea, weak e.g. PG Tips

- White tea
- Fruit and herbal tea, weak – ensure no apple added
- Peppermint tea
- Green tea
- ➢ Water

Dairy Foods and Eggs

- ➢ Butter
- ➢ Cheese:
  - Camembert
  - Brie
  - Cottage – 2 tablespoons
  - Cheddar
  - Feta
  - Cream Cheese – 2 tbsp
  - Haloumi – 40g
  - Goat / chevre
  - Mozzarella
  - Monterey Jack
  - Parmesan
  - Paneer – 2 tbsp
  - Swiss
  - Ricotta – 2 tablespoons
  - Dairy free chocolate pudding

- ➢ Margarine
- ➢ Eggs
- ➢ Milk:
  - Hemp milk – 125ml
  - Almond milk
  - Macadamia milk

- Lactose free milk
- Rice milk
- Oat milk – 30 ml, enough for cereal

- Soy protein (avoid soya beans)
- Sorbet
- Tempeh
- Swiss cheese
- Whipped cream
- Tofu – drained and firm varieties
- Yoghurt:
- Greek yoghurt – 23g
- Coconut yoghurt
- Goats yoghurt
- Lactose free yoghurt

Cooking ingredients, Herbs and Spices

- Oils: Canola oil, Avocado oil, Olive oil, Coconut oil, Rice bran oil, Peanut oil, Soybean oil, Sesame oil, Vegetable oil, Sunflower oil.
- Spices: All spice, Cardamon, Black pepper, Chili powder, Cinnamon, Chipotle chili powder, Cumin, Cloves, Fennel seeds, Curry powder, Goraka, Five spice, Nutmeg, Mustard seeds, Saffron, Paprika, Turmeric, Star anise.
- Herbs: Bay leaves, Basil, Coriander, Cilantro, Fenugreek, Curry leaves, Lemongrass, Gotukala, Oregano, Mint, Parsley, Pandan, Rosemary, Rampa, Tarragon, Sage, Thyme
- Onion infused oil
- Garlic infused oil
- Asafoetida powder – great onion substitute
- Acai powder

- ➤ Baking soda
- ➤ Baking powder
- ➤ Cocoa powder
- ➤ Cacao powder
- ➤ Gelatine
- ➤ Cream, 2 tablespoons
- ➤ Icing sugar
- ➤ Ghee, clarified butter – 1 tbsp
- ➤ Mango Powder – 1 tsp
- ➤ Lard
- ➤ Nutritional yeast
- ➤ Tahini, hulled – 30g
- ➤ Soybean oil
- ➤ Salt

Fodmap Vegetables

LOW FODMAP VEGETABLES

Have you been advised to eat more vegetables over and over again? Do you not know which veggies were considered low FODMAP? It has been demonstratable to eat a number of different vegetables to fulfill our nutritional needs and to eat a variety of herbal foods (including veggies) every week that is good for our intestines. Here is a list of the best low FODMAP plants for your diet.

WHAT IS THE MAJOR VEGETABLE FODMAPS?

Fructans and mannitol are the major FODMAPs found in vegetables. You are probably aware of your FODMAP tolerance levels if you have already completed the FODMAP challenge. In this case, a larger variety of vegetables may be consumed without symptoms of IBS.

Some of the fructans that are strong are: Onion, garlic, artichoke, leek, and spring onion.

Some high in mannitol vegetables include cauliflower, mushrooms, and snow peas.

WHAT ARE LOW FODMAP VEGETABLES?

The following vegetables per 75g served are considered poor in FODMAP.

To primarily include low FODMAP vegetables in order to comply with the recommended five serves of vegetables per day. One serving of vegetables is 75g. This may be 1/2 cup or 1 cup of cooked vegetables.

Low FODMAP vegetable list
- Artichoke
- Alfalfa
- Bean sprouts
- Bamboo shoots
- Bok choy
- Beetroot (pickled)
- Broccolini (stalks only)
- Broccoli (heads)
- Capsicum (red)
- Cucumber
- Cabbage (common)
- Cassava
- Carrot
- Choy Sum
- Chilli (serve = 28g)
- Canned baby corn

- Collard Greens
- Kale
- Edamame
- Lettuce (iceberg, butter, cos)
- Oyster Mushrooms
- Rocket
- Spring onion greens, tops only (serve = 16g)
- Olives
- Potato
- Parsnip
- Radish
- Japanese Pumpkin
- Silver beet
- Rocket
- Spinach
- Spaghetti squash
- Swede
- Squash
- Turnip
- Tomatoes
- Taro

LOW FODMAP 15-MINUTE 5-STEP MEAL PLAN.

Everyone is different, and when it comes to meal preparation, there is no way right. Regardless of whether you cook for one or your whole family, the same rules apply. I have set out a series of steps to follow, which should take approximately 15 minutes per week.

STEP 1: Start the meal planning calendar (1 minute)

Find a recording spot for your meals. You can use your notepad, kitchen calendar, whiteboard, or smartphone. I use the Google Calendar app for my husband on my tablet. Shared access means he can start stuff if I'm not home (maybe a bit of wishful thinking here).

TIP: Record food in a spot where you and other members of the family can see it. Everyone can thus participate in the formation of your low FODMAP meal plan.

STEP 2: Determine how much food you need (1 minute)

The greatest mistake is to think about preparing seven meals a week. It's too overwhelming! See your timetable and decide on which nights to prepare. Here's no wrong response. Some of you may find that two foods are appropriate; others may prefer five meals. The magic number in our household is four. Four dinners can be enjoyed and leave for a few nights and only towing.

TIP: Don't get distracted. Start small and get up to work.

STEP 3: Pick your main (5 minutes)

This is the part people most fear and the exhaustion to decide. Keep it plain, therefore. Use your favorite food and find low swaps in FODMAP. For example: For example:

- Green leek leaves instead of onion
- Gluten free pasta instead of wheat pasta
- Lactose-free dairy instead of lactose-containing dairy.
- Garlic infused oil instead of garlic cloves/powder

These popular swaps will turn many of your favorite foods into your preferred FODMAP meals (and a bit of planning).

Cook easy meals on busy nights. If you have only 30 minutes to prepare dinner, do something fast like a pan dinner or pasta. It's not the night for a complicated and fresh recipe.

Choose a variety of themes. Examples of these include Meatless Mondays, Taco Tuesdays, and Pizza Fridays. Every week you plan a variation on your themes and use again the following week a variation on the same theme. Other potential topics include burgers, fried stir, BBQ, fish, etc.

Do you need inspiration? Look for reliable recipe bloggers (there's a lot of nutritionists!). Cookbooks or online, be suspicious about your source whatever you want. I saw so many "Low FODMAP Recipes" like the FODMAP bombs. Choose sources accredited by, written or updated by, or authorized by, qualified diattians of Monash.

TIP: Click through the Spoonful app's Discovery section to find low FODMAP swaps to see what others scanned. Switch left to save your favorites a meal.

Tips for meal planning:
- Make your favorite food list.
- Use a whiteboard in a kitchen that can be used by your guests.
- Find a low FODMAP cookbook and use your favorite recipes with sticky notes
- Follow Instagram FODMAP specialists and save Instagram recipes.
- Schedule if you have additional time.
- Double your lunch or dinner meals to be saved.
- Set aside time to cook a meal or two on the weekend.

STEP 4: Pick your sides (5 min)

If a man has been selected, it is time to add one or two sides. Strive for half a plate and a fifth of all the grains on your plate. This nutritionist is a big salad fan (I know, so cliche). In the Spoonful app, there are plenty of bag salads and dressings that are easy and convenient. Seek low FODMAP bread, rice, quinoa, gluten-free pasta, and potatoes when selecting grains (with skins on). With a wide range of fibers for goods and whole grains, the gut microbes are helpful. Trust me, and you want these little guys by your side and happy.

TIP: Prepare the bowl of low FODMAP vegetables with carrots, onions, cherry tomatoes, and mini red peppers. Divide them into single portions of scale.

STEP 5: Make your Shopping list

Your last move in the grocery store before setting foot is to make your food list. Write down the ingredients you need and don't forget what you've got.

SPOONFUL TIP: Pick your supermarket by using the filter button. You can check or browse the Discovery section. Swip left to add your favorites to your favorites.

TIP: Divide your list into parts like food, meat, milk, baked goods, etc.

Set it all together

The secret to this work is to prepare your low FODMAP meal before entering the shop. You have so many great choices until you are ready with your chosen meals and your food list. Internet shopping is perfect too because you can find anything you like. Shopping in-store works too. The frequency of your shopping depends on your schedule and the space in your refrigerator. Do the best for you!

Day Low FODMAP Diet Plan For IBS

The 7 days Low FODMAP IBS Meal Plan is a dietary plan for the temporary removal of FODMAPs from your diet that is the reason of irritable bowel syndrome (IBS).

It is designed to give you several ideas and remove your eating plan from your anxiety and devaluation.

Please note that a low FODMAP diet should be strictly followed for at least 28 days (4 weeks). Please first read this to find out why.

After that, it may be period for the reinstatement or task process. Note that your digestive problems can be addressed in other ways than in a low FODMAP diet.

Low FODMAP Diet Plan IBS 7-day

Must-Read Notes Prior to Start:

1. Consult your veterinarian or dietitian first: I do not know your medical history or current prescription or additional factors while changing your diet or exercise regime when I am a certified nutritionist.

2. That meal plan is very stringent and provisional: a low FODMAP diet, not for a medical purpose, is very restrictive. It is also a provisional pattern of food divided into the removal (1st) and replacement (2nd) process – read more. This plan concentrates on the disposal process.

3. Not appropriate for any medical condition: This involves people at risk for eating disorders or nutritional and medical mental fragility; (e.g., type 1 or type 2 diabetes using medication). It is also clear that this is not for children, the diet for the elimination of a child must be monitored by a dietitian directly.

4. Check this Low FODMAP Food List: Size of the serving portion is important since most FODMAP food products still contain small amounts. An apple portion is low in FODMAP, for example, but if you take half an apple in one go, your FODMAP intake will be high. Download this list as a FODMAP Low Food Guide.

5. Water from which to choose: no liquids are included in the food plan, and you can drink and drink a bottle of water. Black tea, black coffee, mint and green tea are very light and okay FODMAP (no milk).

6. To avoid unintentionally eating high food FODMAP typically means preparing food in advance, so I suggest taking the grocery list at the bottom of the post for the weekly recipes.

7. Maintain your food journal: document all meals you have had and if after or after all meals you have had any unwanted symptoms. This is called the food diary and helps you identify causes and reintroduce them later. A mba course of Safe Food Guide NZ, which you can copy or compose on a few papers at houses, can be found here.

8. The often-created recipes make 2-4 chunks: actually, write your shopping list. You're going to have stayed. Feed the family or save another day's food.

9. I strongly recommend you invest $11 in the FODMAP application from Monash University which is accessible on iPhones and Android devices. They have a huge food bank checked for their FODMAP criteria and almost 100 original recettes. A small cost to pay for a lifetime shift.

DAY #1 MONDAY
Breakfast: Low FODMAP Smoothie Blueberry. Make a big batch, so every morning it's ready to leave the fridge.
Low FODMAP Smoothie Blueberry
PREP IN 5 MIN
COOKS IN 1 SECOND
SERVES 1

INGREDIENTS
- 125 ml (1/2 cup) low FODMAP milk*
- Blueberry Smoothie
- 20 blueberries (fresh or frozen)

- 60 ml (1/4 cup) vanilla soy ice cream (or lactose-free ice cream or lactose-free yogurt)*
- 30 g frozen bananas (firm)*
- Six ice cubes
- 1 tsp chia seeds
- 2 tsp rice protein powder*
- 1 tsp lemon juice*
- 1/2 tbsp pure maple syrup (optional)*

Equipment
• blender

DIRECTIONS
Method

FODMAP tips
In a blender, placed low FODMAP milk, frozen blueberries, vanilla soy ice cream (lactose-free ice cream or yogurt). If your frozen banana is in a big chunk, I will encourage you to break it into smaller pieces to make it easier to blend. Fill in the blender with the frozen banana, ice cubes, rice protein powder, chia grains, maple syrup (if used), and lemon juice.

1. Mix until smooth.
2. Serve immediately. Serve immediately. It is best to immediately drink this smoothie. Otherwise, it will melt and split, changing the taste. Note: Peel and cut into 30g (1.06oz) bits before freezing your bananas.

This low FODMAP blueberry smoothie is a perfect way to start your day. Many smoothies that claim they are low in FODMAP also have too many fruit portions for a seat.

We have spent a lot of time making a good smoothie that contains just 1 and 1/3 servings of low safe FODMAP fruit per serving, consistent with the quantity of fruit used by Monash University and Kate Scarlata in their smoothie recipes.

FODMAP Note: Common bananas are FODMAP low in 100g (unripe green or yellow), but they become FODMAP high in fructans when they are ready (yellow with brown spots).

NUTRITION PER SERVE

Fat10.2g, Calories308, Protein5.8g, Saturates1.4g, Sugars30.6g, Carbs49.5g, Salt0.2g, Fibre4.6g, Calcium201.6mg, Iron1.5mg

Lunch: Rice-paper (Fresh Spring) Rolls. Choose from this list a maximum of 3 vegetables, and add the protein if you like. Take out the scallions and avocados.

STEP BY STEP GUIDE TO ROLLING FRESH SPRING ROLLS

PREP TIME15 minutes

TOTAL TIME15 minutes

INGREDIENTS

- 2 large carrots, peeled and sliced julienne style
- 12 rice paper spring roll wrappers
- 1 bell pepper, any color, sliced julienne style
- 1 small zucchini and/or cucumber, sliced julienne style
- 1 avocado, sliced thin
- 1 cup shredded red cabbage
- 1 scallion, green and white parts, chopped
- 2 cups of shredded romaine lettuce
- sauce of choice, I recommend Thai Peanut Sauce
- 1 bunch of cilantros, chopped

DIRECTIONS

1. Before you start, wet your work surface lightly (as this will keep your rice paper wrapper from sticking).

2. Take a single dry rice roll spring wrapper and placed it in a tender, warm water tub. Let the rice paper sit 10-20 seconds in the water or until it's foldable.

3. That's the hard part: keep feeling how flexible the rice paper is. You want to be soft and usable without mushiness.

4. When the rice paper is ready, remove the spring roller wrapper from the water and lay it flat on your wet surface. You're going to want to work hard from here.

5. Place carrot, courgettes, and bell pepper slices in rectangular form from the middle of the wrapper and keep away from the edges of the wrapper.

6. Continue adding all the fillings from purple to cilantro by putting them one by one in the center while retaining the shape of the rectangle in the centre.

7. You don't want your wrapper to break down easily. It's time to shut it when you put all your ingredients in a nice little pile in the middle of the spring roll wrapper!

8. Note: Be careful that your spring roll wrapper is not overfilled, or it will tear the rice paper.

9. Start by folding over the vegetables the top and bottom parts of the rice paper.

110. Starting from the left, scatter around the pile of ingredients on the left side of the wrapper, tuck, and roll until you can rest under the ingredients.

11. Tie the edges in and then roll the spring roll as tightly as possible, without tearing the rice paper wrapper.

12. You just rolled your own spring roll! This is it! Now roll as many spring rolls as you want and eat them right away.

13. Enjoy your favorite sauce for dipping. The Thai Peanut Sauce, Ginger, Soja Sauce, or Coco Aminos, I suggest!

Note: Omit avocado and Low FODMAP scallion diet.
Nutrition Information:
Saturated Fat: 1g; Calories: 240; carbohydrates: 38g; Sodium: 75mg; Sugar: 8g; Fiber: 9g; Protein: 8g

Dinner: Maple Garlic Glazed Salmon + low FODMAP veggies (see link above) + 1 cup of brown rice cooked (for the fiber).
MAPLE GARLIC GLAZED SALMON
INGREDIENTS
- Serves 2-3 people
- 2 tablespoons pure maple syrup
- 1/2-pound salmon filet
- 1 tablespoon soy sauce
- 1 tablespoon garlic infused oil
- Dash of either crushed red pepper or sesame seeds
- Salt and pepper, to taste

DIRECTIONS
1. Preheat 400 degrees F oven
2. Mix maple syrup, soy sauce, garlic-infused milk, salt, and pepper in a small cup.
3. Place salmon in a small glass baker's dish and cover with a mixture of maple and garlic.
4. Marinate for 25-30 minutes in the refrigerator.
5. As asked, sprinkle with broken red pepper or sesame seeds.
6. Bake 20 minutes uncovered in the oven or until flaky and fried.

Snack 1: a huge handful of macadamia, nuts, or walnuts in Brazil (40g maximum). Essential for nutrients and fiber.

Snack 2: Low FODMAP Certified Dark Chocolate, Nuts, and Sea Salt Snack Bar.

DAY #2 TUESDAY

Breakfast: 1/2 cup of rolling oats, ½ banana top, lactose-free milk. More than 1/2 cup of FODMAP is high (oligosaccharides).

Lunch: Kitchen and carrot risotto. This is best prepared in batches in advance.

RECIPES

Low Fodmap Pumpkin & Carrot Risotto

Prep Time - 25 Min

Cooks Time - 35 Min

Serves 4

Ingredients

Roast Veggies

- 240 g (2 large) carrots
- 240 g Japanese pumpkin (Kabocha squash or Buttercup squash)
- Season with salt & pepper
- 1 tbsp olive oil

Risotto

- 40 g (1/2 cup) leek (green tips only)*
- 318 g (1 1/2 cup) medium grain white rice (rice rice)*
- 1 tbsp dairy free spread (olive oil spread or butter) (or olive oil)*
- 1 tbsp garlic infused oil*

- 2 tsp   lemon zest*
- 1000 ml (4 cups)   low FODMAP chicken stock/vegetable stock*
- 120 g (4 cups)   spinach
- 2 1/2 tbsp   lemon juice*
- 50 g   parmesan cheese or vegan parmesan cheese (optional) (grated)*
- 3 tbsp   fresh cilantro (chopped)

DIRECTIONS

1. Preheat the baking feature of the oven to 200oC (390oF). Peel and cut into 1,5cm (0.60 inch) sections the pumpkin and the carrot. In an oven, stir in olive oil and season with salt and pepper. Bake 20-25 minutes (until soft and slightly golden). Toss a few times while cooking.

2. Make the risotto while the roast veggies are cooking. Chop the green leek tips roughly. Make the stock if the stock cubes are used and shred the spinach. Over medium heat, heat a broad casserole. Fry the leek tips in the milk free spread (spread olive oil or butter) and infusion of garlic oil for two minutes. Add the rice and whisk for about 1 minute through the mixture.

3. First, add 125ml (1/2 cup) of stock at a time, stir until fluids have soaked into the rice from time to time. Continue to add and the stir in the stock, splash at a time. Switch heat down to medium-low if necessary (if the rice is cooking too quickly and starting to stick to the bottom of the pan). When about 3/4 of the stock is consumed, check to see if the rice is cooked (should take about 20 minutes). If not, add more stock and continue to cook for a few more minutes. As the risotto cooks, the lemons zest (the trick is just to zest the yellow layer and not the bitter white layer underneath).

4. When the rice is ready to cook, mix the broken spinach, lemon juice, and lemon zest. Season with pepper and salt. Then mix the roast vegetables, new coriander, and rubber cheese (if using).

5. Serve in bowls the pumpkin and carrot risotto. Enjoy! Enjoy!

Nutrition per serve
Calories501; Fat15g; Saturates3.7g; Protein12.4g; Carbs80g; Sugars6.8g; Fibre5.1g; Salt1.4g; Iron2.3mg; Calcium196.1mg

Dinner: Shrimp Brown Rice Noodle & Veggie Stir Fry
RECIPES
Brown Rice Noodle and Veggie Stir Fry with Shrimp
Prep time: 5 mins
Cook time: 30 mins
Total   time: 35   mins
Serves 4 (makes great leftovers!)

INGREDIENTS
- 3 tbsp light brown sugar or maple syrup
- 5 tbsp reduced sodium soy sauce (gluten free if needed)
- 2 tbsp rice vinegar
- 3 tbsp fresh lime juice (1 to 2 limes)
- 1 tbsp vegetable oil
- 2 tsp sesame oil
- 2 cups matchstick carrots
- 1 large red bell pepper, sliced into thin 3-inch strips
- Cooking spray (or additional vegetable oil)
- 1 tbsp chopped fresh ginger (1-inch piece)
- 1 1/4 lb medium shrimp, peeled and deveined
- 5 oz spinach leaves
- Black pepper to taste
- 1/4 tsp salt, plus additional to taste
- 6 scallions, green parts only, sliced
- 8 oz brown rice vermicelli

DIRECTIONS

1. Stir the soy sauce, brown sugar or maple syrup, lime juice, rice vinegar, and sesame oil together in a medium dish. Set aside. Set aside. Heat the vegetable oil medium to high in a large pot. Add the bell peppers and cook, often stirring for approximately 4 minutes. Add carrots and cook until vegetables are crisp, about 4 minutes longer (add a few tablespoons of water to the skillet if vegetables start to stick). Stirring often, add ginger and about 34 of the scallions and cook for 1 minute. Take a medium tub.

2. Return the saucepan to the top of the burner, mist the kitchen spray, and heat on low. Add spinach and then cook for 2 to 3 minutes, frequently stirring until wilted. Apply the carrot mixture to the cup.

3. Return the pot to the stove again and mist the cooking spray (or add more vegetable oil). Medium-high sun. Add to taste shrimp, 1/4 tsp of salt, and black pepper. Cook, turn periodically until shrimp are firm to the touch and opaque, for 4 to 6 minutes, in the thickest region.

4. Carry a big pot of water to a boil in the meantime. Add rice noodles and cook, mix regularly, around 3 minutes. Drain and rinse with cold water in a fine-mesh strainer. Back noodles to the pot in which you cooked them. Give a fast whisk to the soy sauce mixture and apply to the noodles. Heat medium-high and boil. Heat medium-high. Reduce heat to mild, add a mixture of vegetables. Toss gently until mixed and heated. Remove the shrimp. Add salt and pepper to taste and season, if necessary. Serve and garnish with the remaining scallions immediately.

NUTRITION   INFORMATION

Calories: 492 Fat: 9g; Carbohydrates: 68g; Saturated fat: 2g Sodium: 1302mg; Sugar: 14g Protein: 38g; Fiber: 9g

Snack: 1 cup of carrot and cucumber + 3-4 tbsp of cottage cheese. Keep them as a snack or take them to work in the refrigerator.

DAY #3 WEDNESDAY
Breakfast: Banana chocolate oats overnight
Easy One-Pan Ratatouille (Low-FODMAP, gluten free)

Prep time: 5 mins
Cook time: 1 hour
Total   time: 1   hour,   5   mins
Serves 8 (1 serving=1/2 cup)

INGREDIENTS

- 1 med eggplant (1 lb), chopped
- 3 to 4 tbsp olive oil
- 2 small zucchini (12 oz), chopped
- salt and black pepper to taste
- 6 oz thin green beans (haricots verts)
- 1 large red bell pepper (8 oz), chopped
- 3/4 tsp dried herbs (any combo of thyme, tarragon, rosemary, etc)
- 2 1/2 cups unsalted diced tomatoes (from can, jar, etc)
- 1/3 cup chopped olives, such as kalamata
- Red chile flakes or minced fresh red chile (optional)
- Chopped fresh basil
- 4 oz feta cheese, crumbled

DIRECTIONS

1. Heat around the 1 1/2 tbsp of oil on medium heat in a large sauté pan. Add eggplant, salt, black pepper, and constantly cook, stirring until slightly browned (not soft, cooked at this time) for 7 to 10 min. Take a big tub. If any brown bits stick to the pot, add approximately 1/4 cup water (or red wine). When it begins to cool, grind to deglaze the bottom of the pot with a spatula.

2. In the pot, heat approximately 1 1/2 centimes of oil, only medium heat, and add the courgette and bell pepper. Season to finely browned, seven to ten minutes with salt and black pepper. Attach eggplant to the dish. If you like, deglaze the pan again. Apply 1 to 2 tsp of petroleum. Add the green beans and the cook for about 3 minutes, often stirring until lightly browned.

3. Add tomatoes and bring to a frying pan with green beans. Add eggplant, courgettes, bell peppers, dried herbs, and chili flakes if used. Cover and cook over medium to medium-low heat until tender and thickened for 25 to 30 minutes, occasionally stirring. If the pan gets too dry, then add water if necessary before the veggies are done. Remove the olives. Season with salt and black pepper to taste.

4. Serve ratatouille on polenta, pasta, or quinoa without gluten (or use any of the other ideas in this blog post). Feta and new basil sprinkle. I like to add protein chicken.

Nutrition   Information
Calories: 139 Fat: 9g; Carbohydrates: 12g; Saturated fat: 3g Sodium: 296mg; Sugar: 6g Protein: 4g; Fiber: 4g

Lunch: Easy One-Pan Ratatouille
Dinner: Crusted Chicken Parmesan + 1 tablespoon of brown (for fiber) and low FODMAP vegetables Dinner: (from this list). Swap marinara sauce for plain tomatoes tinned.

Quinoa Crusted Chicken Parmesan

INGREDIENTS

- 3-4 chicken breasts, sliced in half and pounded to thin cutlets (about 1 1/2 pounds)
- Serves 4-6; Makes delicious leftovers
- 1/2 cup potato starch
- 1 1/2 cups lactose free milk
- 2 eggs
- salt and pepper, to taste
- 2 teaspoons chopped basil
- 2 cups cooked quinoa
- 1 cup marinara sauce (low FODMAP variety such as Rao's Sensitive Formula)
- 1/4 cup Parmesan cheese
- Fresh sliced basil for garnish if desired
- 1 cup shredded mozzarella cheese

DIRECTIONS

1. To 375 degrees F preheat the oven.
2. Lightly oil broadsheet of the bakery.
3. Add milk and chicken breasts in a medium bowl and set aside.
4. Place the potato starch on the plate and salt and pepper, reserve.
5. Add eggs and whisk in a small bowl, and set aside.
6. Put the quinoa in a bowl and add the basil.
7. Take a cutlet of chicken out of milk and gently dip into the potato starch on both sides, and shake to extract excess starch.
8. Dip the stuffed chicken into eggs and then into quinoa.
9. Push the quinoa tightly into the chicken breast and put the chicken in the pan.
10. Repeat the rest of the chicken process.
11. Parmesan cheese scatter uniformly over chicken breasts.

12. Bake until cooked for 25 minutes.

13. Carefully remove from oven and apply two tablespoons of marinara on each breast and sprinkle with mozzarella. Return to the oven for 5 minutes to melt the cheese and hot sauce; if needed, cover with fresh basil.

Snack 1: 200g (7oz) of yogurt free of lactose
Snack 2: Low FODMAP Certified Almond Coconut Snack Bar.

DAY #4 THURSDAY

Breakfast: Sourdough toast (100% spelt or white wheat) + peanut butter (2 pieces). Learn more about breads here are all right.

Lunch: Quinoa Nuts salad. This recipe has several alternatives depending on the remaining vegetables and nuts. Remove the corn/peas, fruit, asparagus, and cauliflower proposed in the recipe.

Dinner: Low FODMAP Bolognese Spaghetti. You may also use low-certified bolognese FODMAP sauce.

Snack: 1 cup of cottage sticks and carrot + 3-4 tbsp cottage from cottage

DAY #5 FRIDAY

Breakfast: Pick your favorite breakfast.

Lunch: Tomato and Leek Frittata Low-FODMAP

Dinner: Broccoli sesame tofu and walnuts + brown rice (for extra fiber). Brown rice offers extra fiber, but restrict broccoli to 2/3 cup per serving.

Sesame Tofu with Broccoli and Cashews Walnuts or Pine nuts

Sesame Tofu with Broccoli and Cashews Walnuts or Pine nuts

INGREDIENTS
- 2 TB reduced sodium Tamari soy sauce
- 1, 8 oz package extra firm tofu cut in bite size chunks
- 2-3 TB sesame seeds
- 2 tsp. toasted sesame oil
- 1/2-3/4 cup chopped broccoli
- 1-2 TB peanut oil
- 1/4 tsp. dried ginger or 1 tsp finely grated fresh ginger
- 1/4 cup cashews, chopped
- 1 tsp garlic minced, or 2 tsp garlic infused oil

DIRECTIONS

Mix the tofu chunks and sesame oil with soy sauce. Marinate in the refrigerator for 10 minutes to 2 hours.

Drain marinade tofu and position it on a plate. Sprinkle with sesame seeds uniformly.

Add peanut oil and cook over medium heat in a medium skillet.

Add tofu, broccoli, garlic, or chopped garlic and ginger. Cook approximately 2 minutes and stir gently.

Cook until light brown and broccoli are tender for around 4-5 minutes.

For the last minute of cooking, add cashew walnuts or pine nuts.

Snack 1: A huge handful of maize, noodles, or walnuts in Brazil (40g maximum)

Snack 2: 1 small package of corn chips (50 grams) + certified low salsa FODMAP.

DAY #6 SATURDAY
Breakfast: Low FODMAP Pancakes Blueberry.
Lunch: Pick your preference or the remains. Lunch:
Dinner: Pick your favorite / remains / feed
Snack: 200g (7oz) of yogurt free of lactose.

DAY #7 SUNDAY
Breakfast: Sunday Breakfast: Toast poached eggs. Using a deaf toast (white wheat or 100 percent spelt).
Lunch: Pick your favorite meal/residues/food out
Dinner: Korean Bibimbap Nourishing Bowl.
Bibimbap Nourishing Bowl
Prep Time15 mins
Cook Time35 mins
Total Time50 mins

INGREDIENTS
- 1 cup water
- ½ cup brown rice
- 2 cups | 2,65oz | 75g swiss chard without stems OR spinach chopped
- Pinch of salt
- 2,29 oz | 65g courgette julienned
- 2,65 oz | 75g rainbow carrot peeled and julienned
- 6 oz | 170g plain tofu
- 3 tbsp olive oil
- 2 eggs (optional. Omit if vegetarian)
- Pinch of salt
- 1 tbsp | 0,39oz | 11g Sesame seeds optional

- 0,56 oz | 4g green onions green tops only, chopped

DIRECTIONS

1. Put the rice in a saucepot with a pinch of salt and boiling water. Cook at a low temperature until all the water is absorbed and the rice is cooked.

2. Drain and wrap the paper towel in the tofu. Place on top of the tofu a plate and a heavy object and set aside for 15 minutes. This method helps to drain more easily. Cut into medium rectangular strips after pressing the tofu and cover both sides with salt. Grill 5 minutes per side in a hot grill pan or until crispy, golden brown.

3. Simply heat up 2 tbsp of olive oil in a pot for the Swiss Chard, carrots, and zucchini, then sauté the vegetables with salt (one by one) until tender. Chard takes about 5-7 minutes, carrots about 5 minutes, and courgettes 2-4 minutes.

4. Fry the ovens with a tbsp of olive oil (optional) and add a pinch of salt.

5. Top with veggies and tofu and finish with the sunny side of the egg in two bowls.

6. Add green onions and sesame seeds (optional), blend, and serve.

Notes

You can savor a bowl with a traditional bibimbap sauce if desired: 2 - 3 tablespoons FODMAP low red pepper paste + ½ tea cucumber soy-free sauce + 1 tea cucumber apple cidre vinegar + 1 tea cucumber sesame seeds + 1 tea cucumber sesame oil. Mix well and apply the dressing over the bibimbap before mixing.

Snack: Quinoa Muffins Banana Nut. Too many muffins and strong FODMAP.

Banana Nut Quinoa Muffins

Prep Time - 10 Minutes
Cook Time - 20 Minutes
Total Time - 30 Minutes
Serve - 2 Dozen Muffins
INGREDIENTS:
Dry Ingredients

- 1 C quinoa flakes
- 1 & 1/2 C quinoa flour
- 1 Tbsp. cinnamon
- 1/3 C walnuts or pecans, chopped
- 2 tsp. baking soda
- 4 tsp. baking powder
- 1 tsp. salt

Wet Ingredients

- 4 very ripe bananas, mashed
- 4 flax eggs (or 4 real eggs)
- 1/4 C maple syrup
- 1/2 cup almondmilk

Directions:

1. Preheat the oven to 350°F.

2. Next, prepare and gel your flax eggs in the refrigerator.

3. Then combine all dry ingredients in a large bowl. Mixed bananas, almond milk, and maple syrup into a separate smaller bowl and blend in gelled flax eggs.

4. Add wet ingredients to dry and stir until more or less even.

5. In a grated muffin pot, spoon the batter; put it in the oven for 20 minutes. Fork search to verify what is done.

6. Enjoy!

SNACK IDEAS SUGGESTIONS
Additional balanced therapies and snack suggestions...

SNACKS
- Rice crackers + Goat's cheese/Camembert/ small serve brie/feta
- spoonful of peanut butter + Banana slices (half banana)
- Chewy Peanut Butter Cookies
- Egg boiled hard

Desserts and Treats
- •Creamy Coconut Milk Quinoa Pudding
- •Easy Chocolate Chip-Oat Scones
- •Fudgy One-Bowl Brownies
- Zucchini Cups and Cheesy Baked Quinoa

Fodmap Dietary Plan for Relief of Stomach Bloating

Our digestive system addresses our thoughts. That is why we call the stomach the "second brain." If they are agitated or frightened, their bellies will tell them that it's time to calm down in no uncertain terms. Therefore, it is important to know a few basic steps to overcome anxiety, especially a bloated stomach.

The Low Fodmap Dietary Plan
During periods of tension and aggravation, food is sometimes used that feels comfortable but often leads to a bloated belly. It is time to

know what you consume and swap those ingredients for those that are easier in the stomach.

Fodmap are short-chain carbohydrates and body-insufficient alcohols that lead to abdominal pain and bloating.

High Fodmap Foods (Foods to AVOID):
Cashews
Mushrooms
Broccoli, Asparagus, Cauliflower, Peas, Artichokes, Snow Peas, Brussel Sprouts, Beans, Lentils,
Onions
Garlic
Wheat, Rye
Peaches, Apples, Dried Fruits, Pears
Soft Cheeses
Honey
Asparagus
Artichokes
High Fructose Corn Syrup
Wheat- Bread, Pancakes, Pasta

Barley
Products with Lactose: Ice Cream, Custard, Milk, and Yogurt (regular or Greek)
Here are a few foods that will result in reduced digestive symptoms of bloat and discomfort.

Low Fodmap Foods (Good to Eat):
Eggs
Fish
Meats

All Fats and Oils

All Melons, except Watermelon

Blueberries, Bananas, Lemons, Grapes, Oranges, Limes, Strawberries

Hard and Aged Cheeses- Swiss, Cheddar, two soft kinds of cheese only Brie and Camembert.

Vegetables: Celery, Carrots, Green Beans, Cucumbers, Spinach, Potatoes, Zucchini, Tomatoes

Grains such as Oats, Corn, Tapioca, Rice

Beverages: Coffee, Water, Tea

Gelati (instead of ice cream)

Sorbet

Lactose-Free Products

Know sugar substitutes for the same stomach upset and floating, such as sorbitol, xylitol, mannitol. Some gums include counter-medicines, toothpaste, and sugar-free drinks.

Avoid carbonated beverages

Regular activity also helps food digestion and dissipates gas and bloating.

Using a treatment that stops fear by improving the way of thinking and eating.

CONCLUSION

Many people do not know they have IBS before serious symptoms arise. Abdominal discomfort, bloating, diarrhea and constipation may include signs of IBS. These symptoms can weaken and reduce the quality of life. While no known medication for irritable bowel syndrome is available, there are ways to relieve the symptoms.

If you did not understand if you have or do not have IBS, talk to your doctor and registered dietitian nutritionist before you start your "diet" treatment. Meanwhile, here are a couple of tips for help:

Eat Smaller Meals

Large meals may also contribute to clamping and diarrhea of IBS citizens. Eat smaller, then regular meals during the day to prevent this.

Maintain a Food Symptom Diary

The monitoring of food intake, symptoms, and other factors such as stress, medication, everyday activities, and sleep habits helps determine what induces and exacerbates IBS symptoms.

Herbal therapy

Traditional Chinese medicine has been used for a variety of irritable symptoms for thousands of years. Although herbal medicine in America is not widely investigated, clinical trials indicate certain herbs can relieve the frustrating symptoms of IBS. Peppermint oil is supposed to minimize GI tract muscle spasms. Ginger was also used for IBS therapy. Ginger is expected to minimize inflammation, irritation, and nausea.

Try the Probiotics

Several studies indicate that the use of probiotics helps to control the symptoms of IBS. Probiotics are living, microscopic organisms that keep the digestive tract healthy and working properly, called "friendly bacteria" The most popular strains of probiotic bacteria present in yogurt and other cultivated milk products are lactobacilli and bifidobacterium. Often available as food supplements.

Techniques for Stress Relief

While stress did not cause IBS, people with the condition sometimes report increased symptoms in stressful conditions. Measures to minimize stress levels can therefore help with IBS. Consider practices such as meditation, yoga, deep breathing, hypnosis, or guidance. Everyone responds; differently, so different stress reduction methods can need to be tried.

Low FODMAP Diet

If you haven't heard about the low FODMAP diet to treat IBS yet, it's time to look at it. FODMAP is an acronym for the carbohydrate forms that cause annoying effects in the intestines. The sign is the fermentable oligosaccharides, disaccharides, and polyols. These carbohydrates were short-chained and fermented easily by intestinal bacteria. The bacteria which feed on these short-chain carbs develop gas and other unpleasant side-effects that contribute significantly to your comfort. Slowly removing these foods will help you figure out what foods do and do not work for you.

Do not try yourself with a low FODMAP diet. A low FODMAP diet requires an experienced nutritionist who is qualified to use the low FODMAP approach to treat IBS.

Smaller foods, daily dietary symptoms, the use of probiotics, stress reduction, and a low FODMAP diet are all excellent strategies for reducing IBS symptoms. With the support of a licensed dietitian, you will end up on the way to IBS relief by catering for dietary improvements in your way of living.

CPSIA information can be obtained
at www.ICGtesting.com
Printed in the USA
BVHW040947080221
599619BV00006B/127

9 781801 148566